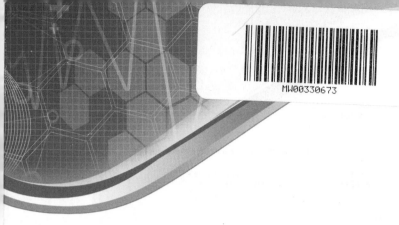

CrossWards
USMLE Step 1 Board Review

Anthony J. Viera, MD, MPH

Associate Professor
Department of Family Medicine
University of North Carolina at Chapel Hill
Chapel Hill, North Carolina

Matthew A. Sutton, MD

Family Medicine Physician
Winslow Indian Health Care Center
Winslow, Arizona

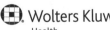 Wolters Kluwer | Lippincott Williams & Wilkins
Health

Philadelphia · Baltimore · New York · London
Buenos Aires · Hong Kong · Sydney · Tokyo

Acquisitions Editor: Susan Rhyner
Product Manager: Catherine Noonan
Marketing Manager: Joy Fisher-Williams
Production Project Manager: Alicia Jackson
Designer: Stephen Druding
Compositor: Aptara, Inc.

Copyright © 2014 Lippincott Williams & Wilkins, a Wolters Kluwer business.

351 West Camden Street
Baltimore, MD 21201

Two Commerce Square
2001 Market Street
Philadelphia, PA 19103

Printed in China

All rights reserved. No part of this book may be reproduced or transmitted in any form or by any means, including as photocopies or scanned-in or other electronic copies, or utilized by any information storage and retrieval system without written permission from the publisher except for brief quotations embodied in critical articles and reviews. To request permission, please contact Lippincott Williams & Wilkins at 2001 Market Street, Philadelphia, PA 19103, via email at permissions@lww.com, or via website at lww.com (products and services).

9 8 7 6 5 4 3 2 1

DISCLAIMER

Care has been taken to confirm the accuracy of the information present and to describe generally accepted practices. However, the authors, editors, and publisher are not responsible for errors or omissions or for any consequences from application of the information in this book and make no warranty, expressed or implied, with respect to the currency, completeness, or accuracy of the contents of the publication. Application of this information in a particular situation remains the professional responsibility of the practitioner; the clinical treatments described and recommended may not be considered absolute and universal recommendations.

The authors, editors, and publisher have exerted every effort to ensure that drug selection and dosage set forth in this text are in accordance with the current recommendations and practice at the time of publication. However, in view of ongoing research, changes in government regulations, and the constant flow of information relating to drug therapy and drug reactions, the reader is urged to check the package insert for each drug for any change in indications and dosage and for added warnings and precautions. This is particularly important when the recommended agent is a new or infrequently employed drug.

Some drugs and medical devices presented in this publication have Food and Drug Administration (FDA) clearance for limited use in restricted research settings. It is the responsibility of the healthcare provider to ascertain the FDA status of each drug or device planned for use in their clinical practice.

To purchase additional copies of this book, call our customer service department at **(800) 638-3030** or fax orders to **(301) 223-2320**. International customers should call **(301) 223-2300**.

Visit Lippincott Williams & Wilkins on the Internet: http://www.lww.com. Lippincott Williams & Wilkins customer service representatives are available from 8:30 am to 6:00 pm, EST.

RRS1306

Puzzled by USMLE preparation or your latest rotation? Tired of the same old boring review? Welcome to *CrossWards*™! We hope you will find these puzzles a more engaging way to review your medical knowledge as you prepare for examinations, ward rotations, or just want to have a fun way to study.

Contributors to this edition of *CrossWards*™ *Step 1*:
Meredith Gilliam, MD, MPH, internal medicine resident at the University of Michigan.
Yemeng Lu, medical student at the University of North Carolina at Chapel Hill School of Medicine.

Look for *CrossWards*™ *Step 2* and other future editions of *CrossWards*™!

Do YOU want to contribute to an upcoming edition of *CrossWards*™? Send your puzzle clues, solutions, and "extra info" in an Excel or Word table (or a Clinical Scramble as a Word file) to: crosswards.submit@gmail.com. We'd also love to receive your other ideas for puzzles! Include your name, address, and current position/medical school. We will let you know if your puzzle is selected for inclusion in an upcoming edition.

PUZZLES

CrossWard Solutions (with a little extra info!) begin on page 102.

1 My Heart Skips a Beat (when I do this puzzle)

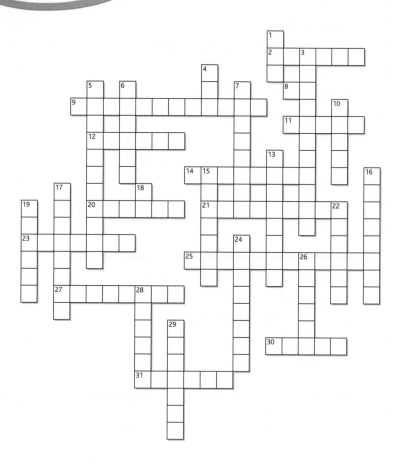

Across:

2 - Cardiac conduction velocity is slowest through this

8 - Classic ECG finding of acute MI: _____ segment elevation

9 - Carotid massage works via a _____ to decrease heart rate

11 - This organ receives the largest share of cardiac output

12 - Stroke volume × heart rate = cardiac _____

14 - Beriberi, which can cause dilated cardiomyopathy, is due to the deficiency of this

20 - Fixed splitting of the second heart sound occurs in atrial _____ defect

21 - Depolarization occurs when there is an influx of this into the myocardial cells

23 - Ventricular action potential plateau is due to an influx of _____

25 - Irregularly irregular rhythm with no discernible P waves = atrial _____

27 - Harsh crescendo–decrescendo systolic murmur could signify aortic _____

30 - Systolic pressure – diastolic pressure = _____ pressure

31 - This valve closes during the first heart sound (S1)

Down:

1 - Cardiac muscle cells are coupled each other by these junctions

3 - Atrial _____ peptide is released when the atria "stretch" in response to increased volume

4 - 1/3 systolic pressure + 2/3 diastolic pressure (acronym)

5 - Hormone that promotes water retention and direct arteriolar vasoconstriction

6 - The dicrotic notch of the cardiac cycle represents closure of the _____ valve

7 - Autoregulation keeps blood flow to an organ _____

10 - Pulmonary capillary _____ pressure measured with a catheter provides an estimate of left atrial pressure

13 - Cardiac relaxation phase

15 - _____ causes vasodilation in all organs except the lungs, where it causes vasoconstriction

16 - Cardiac conduction velocity is fastest through these fibers

17 - The murmur of mitral valve _____ is described as a systolic crescendo murmur with a midsystolic click

18 - Contraction of the left ventricle occurs during the _____ interval

19 - A patent _____ arteriosus may be due to prematurity or congenital infection

22 - Progressive lengthening of PR interval until a beat (QRS) is dropped: _____ type I second-degree block

24 - This biomarker of MI lasts about 10 days

26 - P-wave = _____ depolarization

28 - The ventricular action potential begins when voltage-gated _____ channels open

29 - Cardiac contraction phase

2 A Bug's Life 1

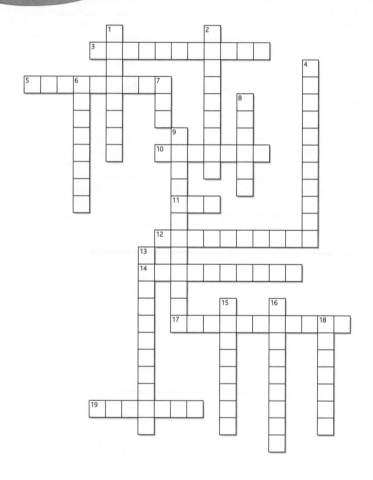

Across:

3 - If your febrile patient returning from South America has "black vomit" and jaundice, think this virus (two words)

5 - Hand-foot-and-mouth disease is caused by _____ virus type A

10 - Protozoan genus that causes watery diarrhea

11 - Major cause of viral pneumonia in infants (initials)

12 - _____ B19 causes erythema infectiosum (fifth disease)

14 - Antibiotic-associated diarrhea is usually caused by the toxin from this organism (genus first letter and species)

17 - Fluke associated with bladder cancer (genus)

19 - Human herpesvirus (HHV)-6 causes this infantile illness

Down:

1 - This cell membrane acid is unique to gram-positive organisms

2 - A person with cough, fever, night sweat, and weight loss due to tuberculosis has this form

4 - Its toxin leads to gas gangrene: Clostridium _____ (species)

6 - One of the oxidase negative, lactose nonfermenting gram-negative rods (genus)

7 - Responsible for classic mononucleosis (initials)

8 - Bats, raccoons, and skunks, oh my! This CNS infection has high fatality rate

9 - Hepatitis A belongs to this virus family

13 - Gram-positive rods in branching filaments that resemble fungi and form sulfur granules (genus)

15 - Shigella inactivates the 60S one of these

16 - Major cause of infant diarrhea around the world and winter daycare diarrhea in US

18 - If you see trophozoites and schizonts on a patient's blood smear, think _____

Solutions on page 105.

3 A Rate-limiting Puzzle

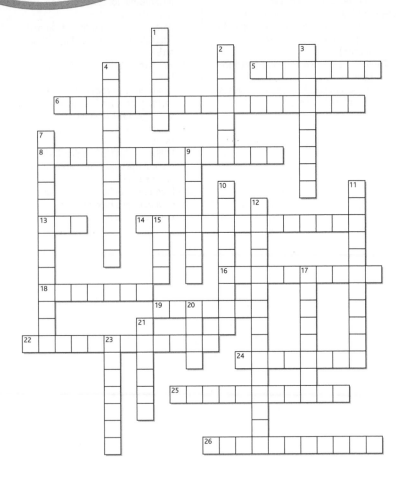

Across:

5 - Stunted growth and cachexia in children due to prolonged deficiency of protein and calories

6 - The rate-determining enzyme of glycolysis

8 - Byproducts of fatty acid metabolism, acetone can be detected in urine but this ketone body cannot: Beta-_____

13 - G6PD is the rate-limiting step in the _____ shunt (initials)

14 - Enzymes that stimulate release of arachidonic acid from phospholipids

16 - _____ dehydrogenase is the rate-limiting step of the tricarboxylic (citric) acid cycle

18 - Pyruvate is converted to this acid by dehydrogenase

19 - Primary source of energy for your brain (Hint: Not caffeine)

22 - Lipoxygenase acting on arachidonic acid results in these compounds

24 - When DNA has had a rough day and it just needs to unwind, it relies on this (Hint: Not a glass of wine)

25 - HMG-CoA synthase is the rate-limiting step in _____

26 - One of four enzymes required for #12 down: Glucose-6-_____

Down:

1 - _____ reductase regulates cholesterol synthesis (acronym)

2 - Rare disease due to the deficiency of glucocerebrosidase

3 - Rate-limiting step of fatty acid metabolism is the _____ shuttle

4 - Substrate in the rate-limiting step in gluconeogenesis: Fructose-1,6-_____

7 - Glycogen _____ is the rate-limiting step of glycogenolysis

9 - The receptor for insulin is part of a large family of _____ kinase receptors

10 - A noncompetitive _____ has no effect on substrate binding and therefore, no effect on Km

11 - Homocystinuria is caused by the deficiency of this synthase

12 - De novo synthesis of glucose

15 - ALA synthase is the rate-limiting step in _____ synthesis

17 - Deficiency of hexosaminidase A leads to this disease

20 - Carbamoyl phosphate synthetase I is the rate-limiting step of this cycle

21 - This enzyme seals the DNA deal

23 - Cleaves peptide bonds on the carboxyl side of lysine or arginine

Solutions on page 107.

4 How Many Psychiatrists Does it Take...?*

Yemeng Lu**

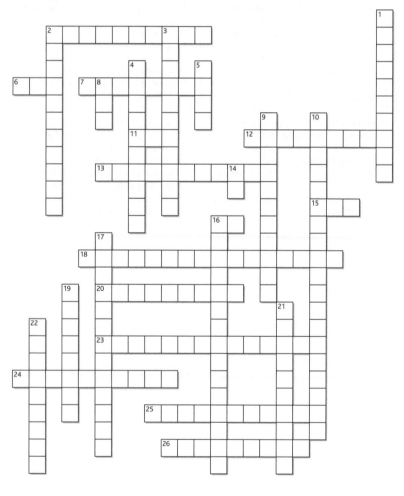

Across:

2 - Chronic factitious disorder: _____ syndrome

6 - Treatment of panic disorder that addresses dysfunctional emotions and maladaptive behaviors (acronym)

7 - "A" in SIG E CAPS stands for _____

11 - A sensitive indicator of alcohol use (laboratory marker, acronym)

12 - Antidepressant that girls on the eating disorder unit should avoid

13 - High-potency neuroleptic known for causing EPS

15 - Treatment of choice for refractory major depressive disorder with the major adverse side effect being amnesia (acronym)

16 - The tried-and-true best relapse prevention for alcohol dependence (acronym)

18 - Symptoms similar to schizophrenia, but for only 3 months

20 - Antidepressant known to cause priapism

23 - Low-potency antipsychotic associated with corneal deposits

24 - Your patient on a neuroleptic develops a fever, muscle rigidity, has unstable vitals and myoglobinuria. You treat with _____

25 - Milder form of bipolar disorder characterized by dysthymia and hypomania: _____ disorder

26 - Defense mechanism that borderline patients use: Believing that people are either all good or all bad

Down:

1 - Treatment for benzodiazepine overdose

2 - Antidepressant of choice for little old ladies who need to sleep better and gain weight

3 - Think hard! You probably have a friend who has very odd beliefs about magic powers, has eccentric behaviors, and is socially awkward; he most likely has _____ personality disorder

4 - MAO-B inhibitor used in Parkinson disease

5 - Stereotyped hand-wringing in a previously healthy 4-year-old girl who can no longer speak: _____ syndrome

8 - Intoxication with _____ produces impulsiveness, belligerence, nystagmus, psychosis (acronym)

9 - A CEO of a large bank who is frustrated at work and releases his energy in the gym demonstrates a defense mechanism called _____

10 - The psychiatrist who gets upset at the patient for substance abuse because his own mother recently passed away from alcoholic liver cirrhosis is exhibiting _____

14 - A severe alcohol withdrawal (acronym)

16 - Your patient on clozapine requires weekly WBC monitoring to check for _____

17 - The neurotransmitter thought to be decreased in Alzheimer dementia

19 - One out of five patients with this syndrome has coprolalia

21 - Jimmy is 12 and still wets the bed and has failed the bed alarm; let us try this medication

22 - pH disturbance in bulimia nervosa patients: Metabolic _____

*to change a light bulb?
  Answer: only one, but the light bulb has to want to change.
**Yemeng Lu was a third-year medical student at the University of North Carolina at Chapel Hill at the time of this contribution.

5   What's the Antidote?

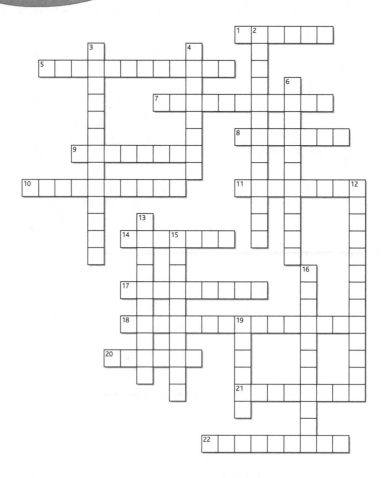

Across:

1 - Induces vomiting: Syrup of _____
5 - Iron toxicity
7 - Used with #21 across
8 - Methanol ingestion
9 - Beta-blocker toxicity
10 - Benzodiazepine overdose
11 - Amphetamine toxicity: _____ chloride
14 - Kit for this poisoning includes amyl nitrite and thiosulfate
17 - Reverses heparin
18 - Acetaminophen overdose
20 - 1-800-222-1222: _____ control number in US
21 - Insecticide (organophosphate) poisoning
22 - Anti-dig Fab fragments are used for toxicity from this

Down:

2 - Anticholinergic toxicity
3 - Copper toxicity
4 - Reverses warfarin
6 - Aspirin overdose: Sodium _____
12 - Methemoglobin (two words)
13 - CO poisoning: _____ oxygen
15 - Opiate overdose
16 - Mercury toxicity
19 - Rattlesnake bite (trade name)

6 Your Microtubules are Showing

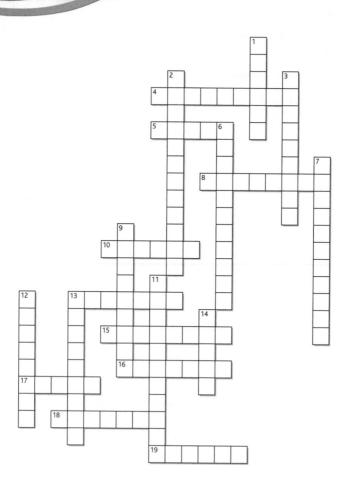

Across:

4 - Kinds of bonds important to maintain #8 across
5 - Form of endoplasmic reticulum; that is, the site of synthesis of secretory proteins
8 - Final structure of most proteins is the _____ structure
10 - Muscle cell stain
13 - Term for complete failure of cell production
15 - Irreversible cell injury/death
16 - Microtubules are made up of dimers of alpha- and beta-_____
17 - Rb and p53 are _____ suppressors
18 - Consists of prophase, metaphase, and anaphase
19 - Form of endoplasmic reticulum; that is, site of steroid synthesis

Down:

1 - Rapidly dividing cells that never go to G_0
2 - When these are damaged, cytochrome c and H+ are released
3 - Phase missing from clue #18 across
6 - Increase in the size of an organ due to an increase in the size of the cells
7 - Increase in the size of an organ due to an increase in the number of cells
9 - Cells that stay in G_0 and regenerate from stem cells
11 - Collagen-making cells
12 - Connective tissue stain
13 - Programmed cell death
14 - These have a 9 + 2 arrangement of microtubules

Solutions on page 113.

7 Where is My Mind?

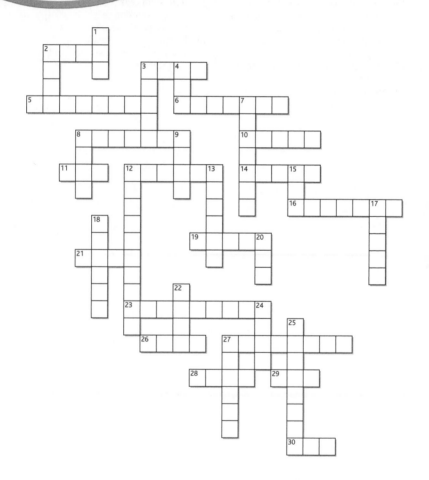

Across:

2 - Herniation of L4–L5 disc would produce a L _____ radiculopathy
3 - High-frequency cochlea
5 - Fascicle of the lower limb
6 - Site of decussation: Posterior columns
8 - Site of decussation: Corticospinal tract
10 - Unilateral hemianopsia lesion: Optic _____
11 - _____ encephalon (forms pons/cerebellum)
12 - Bitemporal hemianopsia lesion: Optic _____
14 - _____ encephalon (hindbrain)
16 - Myelinator cell
19 - Cranial nerve assessed by gag reflex
21 - _____ encephalon (forebrain)
23 - Unilateral quadrantanopia lesion: Optic _____
26 - Low-frequency cochlea
27 - Fascicle of the upper limb
28 - _____ mater: Outermost layer of meninges
29 - _____ mater: Innermost layer of meninges
30 - Cranial nerve for pupils

Down:

1 - _____ encephalon (forms cerebral hemispheres)
2 - Superior oblique cranial nerve
3 - Plate of neural tube that forms motor nerves
4 - Muscle innervated by CN XI
7 - Geniculate body for light
8 - _____ encephalon (forms medulla)
9 - Plate of the neural tube that forms sensory nerves
12 - Site of decussation: Spinothalamic tract
13 - Geniculate body for music
15 - _____ encephalon (midbrain)
17 - Unilateral blindness lesion: Optic _____
18 - Herniation of this part of the cerebellum seen in Arnold–Chiari malformation
20 - Longest cranial nerve in the brain
22 - Herniation of C4–C5 disc would produce a C _____ radiculopathy
24 - Taste to the posterior third of the tongue by this cranial nerve
25 - Upper motor neuron "sign"
27 - Macular sparing lesion: Optic _____

Solutions on page 115.

8 Ain't Life Gland?

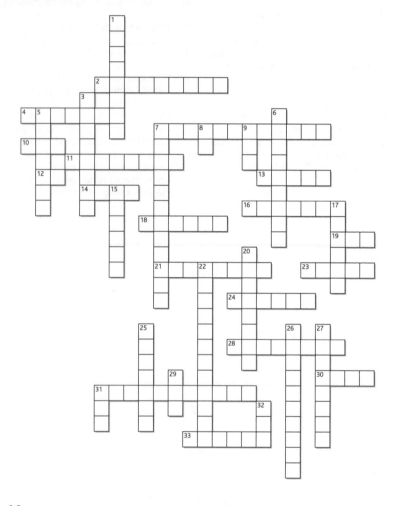

Across:

2 - #31 across also increases renal secretion of this electrolyte
4 - Thyroglossal duct cysts are found midline or lateral
7 - Responsible for breast development during puberty
10 - Promotes growth of ovarian follicle (acronym)
11 - Systemic anti-inflammatory effects, immunosuppression, elevation of blood glucose
12 - Triggers ovulation
13 - #31 down increases reabsorption of this molecule in the distal tubule
14 - Triggers LH/FSH release (acronym)
16 - Branchial cleft cysts are found midline or lateral
18 - #21 across stimulates contractions of this smooth muscle organ
19 - Stimulates release of thyroid hormone
21 - Stimulates milk letdown
23 - _____ corticoids are released from adrenal cortical zona fasciculata
24 - Testosterone is produced in these cells in the testes
28 - Pancreatic hormone which increases blood glucose
30 - Promotes secretion of adrenal cortical hormones
31 - Increases renal retention of Na^+
33 - LH acts on these cells in testes and increases testosterone production

Down:

1 - Causes proliferation of endometrium
3 - Congenital absence of the parathyroids may be seen in this syndrome
5 - Pancreatic hormone which decreases blood glucose
6 - Stimulates milk production
7 - Promotes transition from proliferative to secretory endometrium
8 - Promotes increase in lean body mass
9 - Promotes release of TSH from the thyroid and prolactin from the anterior pituitary
15 - Craniopharyngioma forms from the remnants of this embryologic pouch
17 - LH promotes formation of the corpus _____
20 - _____ corticoids are released from adrenal cortical zona glomerulosa
22 - Triggers spermatogenesis
25 - FSH acts on these cells to promote sperm maturation
26 - "Tones down" calcium in the blood
27 - Inhibits prolactin release
29 - Increases serum calcium, "trashes phosphate"
31 - Causes constriction of vascular smooth muscle through its V1 receptor
32 - Maintains the corpus luteum if implantation occurs

Solutions on page 117.

9   Clinical Scramble

LORIPAUY

RUGBYDIEL

GAPYOLIPHA

TENMORFIM

OPLIDAYSIP

ANSWER: _____

Notes

10 Let's Get PUMPED!

Yemeng Lu*

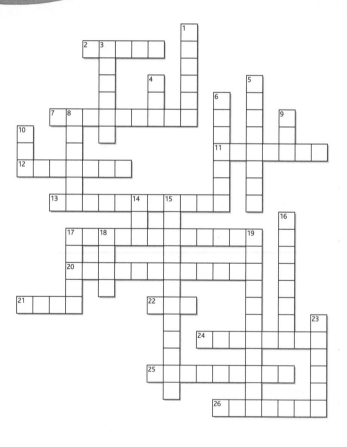

*Yemeng Lu was a third-year medical student at the University of North Carolina at Chapel Hill at the time of this contribution.

Across:

2 - Enlargement of the left atrium can produce hoarseness due to the compression of a nerve; that is, a branch of the _____ nerve

7 - Fetal vessel with the highest oxygenation: _____ vein

11 - A pregnant 25-year-old woman with well-controlled bipolar type I mood disorder is at risk for having a child with _____ anomaly of the heart

12 - Medication that works by inhibiting Na/K ATPase and increases cardiac contractility

13 - _____ can be associated with familial hypercholesterolemia and cholesterol deposited underneath the skin of the eyelid

17 - The murmur of _____ cardiomyopathy increases with the Valsalva maneuver

20 - Your patient who works at a plastic manufacturing company producing vinyl products is at risk for developing _____

21 - Tetralogy of fallot will likely result in a _____ -shaped cardiac silhouette

22 - The most common congenital cardiac anomaly (acronym)

24 - IVIG (which evidently can cost $10,000) + aspirin is the treatment of choice for kids with _____ disease

25 - Treatment of choice for a patient with ventricular tachy with shifting sinusoidal waveforms on ECG

26 - These lesions are nontender, erythematous, macular/nodular on the palm and soles and pathognomonic for infective endocarditis

Down:

1 - The QRS complex in ECG corresponds to the closing of the _____ valve

3 - Your patient unintentionally bobs his head with every heartbeat; he likely has pathology in his _____ valve (P.S. There is no "Call Me Maybe" playing in the room)

4 - Embryonic structure: Right common cardinal vein and right anterior cardinal vein give rise to the _____ (acronym)

5 - Your 65-year-old patient, 4 weeks post an acute-MI presents with sudden, sharp, pleuritic, and positional chest pain likely has _____ syndrome

6 - A continuous machine-like murmur heard in an infant can result from congenital _____ infection

8 - "Ball-valve" obstruction in the left atrium

9 - For babies with transposition of the great artery, this agent can be used to keep a fetal vessel open in order to improve oxygenation (acronym)

10 - Artery that supplies the apex and anterior septum of the heart (acronym)

14 - This inflammatory marker is often elevated in patients with temporal arteritis (acronym)

15 - You hear a split S2 sound that does not vary with respiration in a child and suspect _____ defect (two words)

16 - You tell a patient, "Bear down like you are having a bowel movement (but DON'T!)" to perform the _____ maneuver

17 - This organ is super efficient in extracting O_2 – 100% and has largest arteriovenous O_2 difference

18 - The pathogenesis of atherosclerosis involves migration of the smooth muscle cell which is influenced by the mitogen/chemoattractant _____ (acronym)

19 - Your 48-year-old patient who has BP of 160/90 on the right arm and 170/92 on the left arm and has no peripheral pedal pulses likely has _____ of the aorta

23 - Approximate pulse pressure of a patient with a diastolic BP of 60 and MAP of 90

11 A Short Round of Chemo (Drugs)

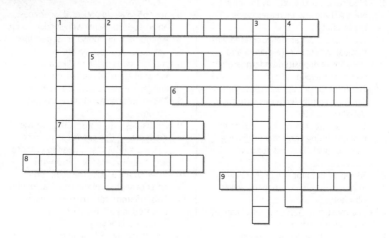

Across:

1 - Alkylating agent used to prevent transplant rejection as well as for some cancers

5 - Alkylating agent used for leukemia; classic toxicity is pulmonary fibrosis

6 - 5-_____ is a pyrimidine analog that binds folate, used topically to treat basal cell carcinoma

7 - Competitively binds estrogen receptors, used to treat estrogen-receptor + breast cancers

8 - Depolymerizes microtubules so spindle cannot form

9 - Trade name Gleevec, this tyrosine kinase inhibitor is used to treat CML

Down:

1 - Another alkylating agent, used for bladder cancer, can damage the acoustic nerves

2 - Given as a rescue medication to reverse bone marrow suppression

3 - Dihydrofolate reductase inhibitor used to treat leukemia/lymphoma, rheumatoid arthritis, psoriasis, and even ectopic pregnancy

4 - Used for Hodgkin lymphoma and myeloma, this agent's classic adverse effect is cardiotoxicity (leading to heart failure)

Solutions on page 123.

12 GI Know that Part

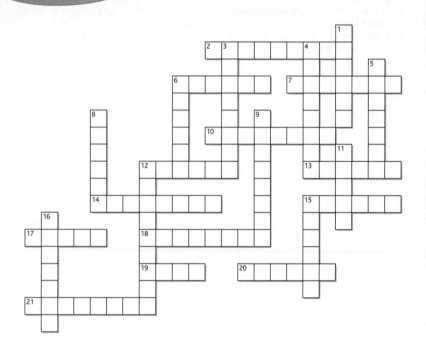

Across:

2 - Divides upper and lower anal canal: _____ line

6 - The _____ duct combines with the common hepatic duct to form the common bile duct

7 - Hernia below the inguinal ligament lateral to pubic tubercle

10 - Hesselbach triangle is formed by the inferior epigastric artery, the _____ ligament, and the lateral border of the rectus abdominis

12 - This cranial nerve courses through the parotid

13 - If your stomach is riding up through your diaphragm, you have a _____ hernia

14 - Proximal one-third of esophagus is composed of this type of muscle

15 - The ligament of _____ connects fourth part of the duodenum to the diaphragm near the splenic flexure

17 - Lymphoid tissue in the lamina propria of small intestine: _____ patches

18 - Direct hernia passes medial to the _____ epigastric artery

19 - Regulates release of bile into the duodenum: Sphincter of _____

20 - The superior mesenteric vein and splenic vein join to form the _____ vein

21 - The gastroduodenal artery is just posterior to the first part of this

Down:

1 - #11 down opens into the _____ part of the duodenum

3 - The _____ anal sphincter is composed of striated muscle

4 - Enteric plexus between the longitudinal and circular layers of GI tract

5 - "Walls" in the colon

6 - This artery, via branches off its trunk, supplies blood to stomach, liver, gallbladder, pancreas, and spleen

8 - This vein runs up the right side of the thoracic vertebral column providing an alternate path for blood to get into the right atrium (e.g., if IVC is blocked)

9 - This branch of the abdominal aorta comes off at L1: _____ mesenteric artery

11 - The pancreatic duct and common bile duct empty into the duodenum through the ampulla of _____

12 - Ligament that connects liver to anterior abdominal wall

15 - The three longitudinal bands of smooth muscle in the large intestine: _____ coli

16 - Where you will find your plicae circulares (if you look hard enough)

13 Private Parts

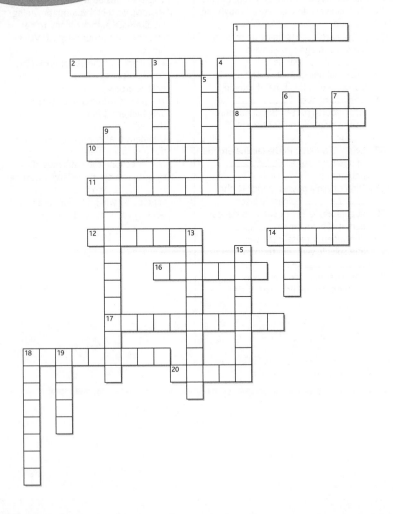

Across:

1 - Sperm are stored in these prior to ejaculation: _____ vesicles
2 - Finger-like projections at the opening of the fallopian tubes
4 - These run from the uterine fundus to the labia majora: _____ ligaments
8 - Distal 1/3 of genital lymphatic drainage is via the superficial _____ nodes
10 - Uterine vessels are contained in this ligament
11 - Pair of sponge-like regions of erectile tissue within the penis dorsally: Corpus _____
12 - Portion of uterine tube that is usual site of fertilization
14 - Membranous layer of superficial fascia of penis: _____ fascia
16 - Longest segment of uterine (fallopian) tubes
17 - Inner lining of the uterus
18 - Layer of connective tissue covering the testicles: Tunica _____
20 - The left testicle's venous drainage is from the left gonadal vein to the left _____ vein

Down:

1 - Urethra runs through the corpus _____ of the penis which also forms the glans
3 - Ureter is posterior and _____ to uterine artery
5 - Spermatogenesis occurs in the semi-niferous _____
6 - Everyone's favorite embryonic structure, this aids in the descent of the gonads
7 - The serous covering of the testes: Tunica _____
9 - Erection is enabled by the _____ nervous system
13 - Normal position of uterus
15 - Ovary epithelium is simple _____
18 - Regressed form of the corpus luteum: Corpus _____
19 - This "ligament" connects the uterus, uterine tubes, and ovaries to the pelvic side wall

Solutions on page 127.

14 This Puzzle Makes My Brain Hurt

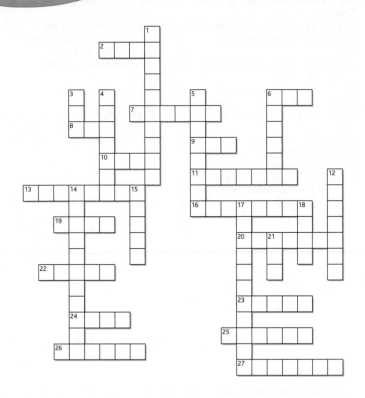

Across:

2 - Artery (acronym): L hemiparesis, L facial droop, L sided neglect
6 - Most common cause of mental retardation (acronym)
7 - Syndrome of ptosis, anhidrosis, flushing, miosis
8 - Debilitating disease of upper and lower motor neurons (acronym)
9 - "Wacky, wobbly, and wet" disease (acronym)
10 - Artery (acronym): R homonymous hemianopsia
11 - Indicates that a seizure lead to loss of consciousness
13 - Hematoma with a concave shape
16 - Hematoma with a lucid interval
19 - A subarachnoid hemorrhage may be seen in patients with this disease (acronym)
20 - Multiple sclerosis triad of nystagmus, scanning speech, intention tremor
22 - Toxin that wrinkles ACh release
23 - Form of expressive aphasia
24 - Cardiac arrhythmia responsible for majority of cardioembolic stroke (short form)
25 - Cranial nerve affected in Bell's palsy
26 - Imaging study obtained STAT with any suspected stroke
27 - Most common mechanism of stroke

Down:

1 - Marching seizure (or perhaps moonwalking?)
3 - "Clot busting" drug indicated for some strokes (acronym)
4 - Artery: Drop attack and vertigo
5 - Form of fluent aphasia, sometimes a "word salad"
6 - Women need adequate quantities of this vitamin to prevent neural tube defects
12 - Artery: Amaurosis fugax
14 - Posturing characterized by flexion
15 - Artery (acronym): L facial sensory loss, R body sensory loss
17 - Posturing characterized by extension
18 - Artery (acronym): R hemiparesis, R facial droop, aphasia
21 - Serum marker elevated in neural tube defects (acronym)

Solutions on page 129.

15 FOOSH!*

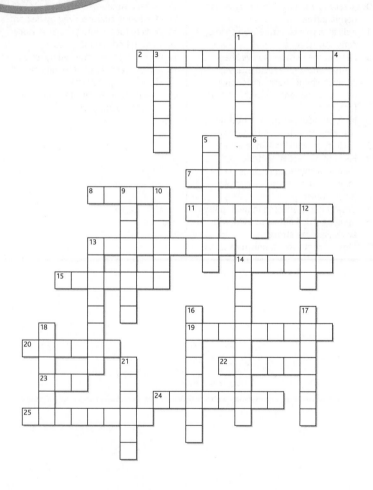

*Fall on outstretched hand – a common mechanism of injury.

Across:

2 - When standing on one leg, the opposite hip drops: _____ sign
6 - Distal radius fracture with dorsal displacement of hand
7 - Fracture of the fifth metacarpal is also known as a _____ fracture
8 - Injury to _____ trunk of brachial plexus can lead to waiter's tip
11 - Jumping off your roof might cause you to fracture one
13 - Lateral curvature of spine
14 - Ability to plantar flex our foot is courtesy of the _____ nerve
15 - A positive #2 across can indicate injury to superior _____ nerve
19 - An overlooked scaphoid fracture can result in _____ necrosis
20 - One of the 6 P's of compartment syndrome
22 - If you just fell down while doing this puzzle and fractured your clavicle, the most likely site is the _____ one-third
23 - Positive anterior drawer test = torn _____ (acronym)
24 - Tenderness in #13 down after a fall on an outstretched hand suggests _____ fracture
25 - _____ paresthetica can result from injury to lateral femoral cutaneous nerve

Down:

1 - Covers the median nerve: _____ retinaculum
3 - Artery that runs through #13 down
4 - One for the gunners: The ulnar nerve runs through this canal
5 - Damage to long _____ nerve can result in winged scapula
6 - #21 down = _____ tunnel syndrome
9 - Foot drop can result from damage to common _____ nerve
10 - Damaged _____ nerve could lead to wrist drop
12 - Damaged _____ nerve could lead to claw hand
13 - Area bordered by ligaments of extensor pollicis longus, extensor pollicis brevis, and abductor pollicis longus
14 - The only one of the rotator cuff muscles that will fit in this spot of the puzzle
16 - This wrist bone sits on the scaphoid and lunate
17 - Tennis elbow = _____ epicondylitis
18 - This wrist bone comes with a hook
21 - Entrapment of _____ nerve leads to paresthesias in thumb, index, and middle finger

Solutions on page 131.

16 A Puzzle to Earn Immunity

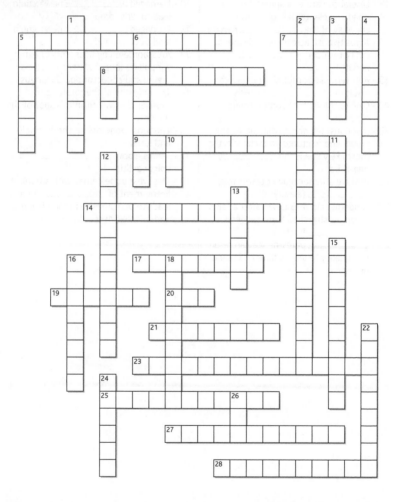

Across:

5 - Determines antibody's antigen specificity: _____ region
7 - Macrophages, neutrophils, and natural killer cells are part of our _____ immunity
8 - CD4+ T-cells make gamma-_____
9 - Primary biliary cirrhosis: Anti _____ antibodies
14 - Antibody to basement membrane: _____ syndrome
17 - Stain used to spot amyloid (two words)
19 - Small molecule that can be antigenic when attached to a carrier
20 - First class of immunoglobulin produced upon antigenic exposure
21 - Hereditary angioedema is caused by the deficiency of C1 _____ inhibitor
23 - Autoimmune connective tissue disorder characterized by heliotrope rash
25 - Vasodilator that can cause a lupus-like syndrome
27 - Check these antibodies if you suspect celiac sprue
28 - This type of cell has major histocompatibility complex issues! Class II that is

Down:

1 - Live attenuated vaccines induce this type of active immune response
2 - HLA-B27 disease (two words)
3 - Two Fab fragments and an Fc results when this "does its thing" on an immunoglobulin
4 - c-ANCA: _____ granulomatosis
5 - B lymphocytes are major cells of the _____ immune response
6 - Therapy used for non-Hodgkin lymphoma, it is an antibody to CD20
8 - Immunoglobulin in breast milk
10 - Mediates septic shock: _____ -alpha (initials)
11 - Anti-dsDNA and anti-Smith, think _____ (short form)
12 - Fancy word for binding bacteria done by C3b
13 - Antibodies to the thyroid-stimulating hormone receptor: _____ disease
15 - Part of the lymph node that is home to Mr. T cells
16 - HLA-DR3: Type 1 _____
18 - Problems with complement pathway C5b to C9 may lead to recurrent infections by this genus
22 - IgE causes its release from mast cells and basophils
24 - A 22q11 deletion leads to failure of this to develop, leading to recurrent viral infections
26 - Most abundant type of immunoglobulin

Solutions on page 133.

17 Bug Hunt

```
G Y E R S I N I A P E S T I S Z T H Y Q G N
O C N I U K C U F J A X W S U E R W N C V T
T S D B C R M Y C O B A C T E R I A Q X Y K
T W O O C R Y E L L O W F E V E R B E T A T
G J T S O R S I P S E U D O M O N A S M C U
E C O O C O T U S A H U K C Q I P C E S T P
V Y X M O T R Z R L S O S M M X T I V P I E
P M I E L A E A A I T T I N J B X T H G N A
E X N T Y V P I B N V E E A C Y A R R O O X
R T B S H I T R C I C A J U T P C A V L M P
F K Z S P R O S I H E K N V R I W C V O Y X
R X E Q A U C V S O O S F R G E R I C T C G
I D I D T S O K T Z N I K S O C L N V X E L
N C O X S A C K I E W S C B A C I L L U S L
G Q E U I Z C D I F F I C I L E I A A S C Y
E Z L W O Q I Y R A D N O C E S G P F C H F
N Y S C W E G S S E G P Y P H Z S L X P I Y
S R A C J D D H H U Z A C M T A C S X Y S D
J U K P E N I V I P R L L C M O N C U O T Z
J B Y Q F X T X G E X I E A R A C C V P O T
X F H E F O R D E M Q S V Z C O L H R T S X
Y R H C E Z V W L B Z T M O F T S T I E O Q
X D R V H D D O L X V E K H V O I E O N M Z
N Q M O B H N M A L A R I A M R Q A O S A D
Z Q J X B B I Z X T G I A R D I A A E L E N
B B B P A P I L L O M A V I R U S P M M A D
E N G H M X J E U J M R I A A R L H G B K U
N N A D E N Y L A T E C Y C L A S E N S P I
```

Actinomyces	Adenylate cyclase	Agalactiae
Bacillus	Bacitracin	Beta
C difficile	Chancre	Coxsackie
EBV	Endotoxin	Giardia
Listeria	Malaria	Maltose
Mycobacteria	Nucleus	Optochin
Papillomavirus	Parvovirus	Pasteurella
Perfringens	Picornavirus	Prions
Pseudomonas	Rabies	Ribosome
Roseola	Rotavirus	RSV
Schistosoma	Secondary	Shigella
Staphylococcus	Streptococci	Teichoic
Tzanck	Yellow fever	Yersinia pestis

18 For Old Timers' Sake

Meredith Gilliam*

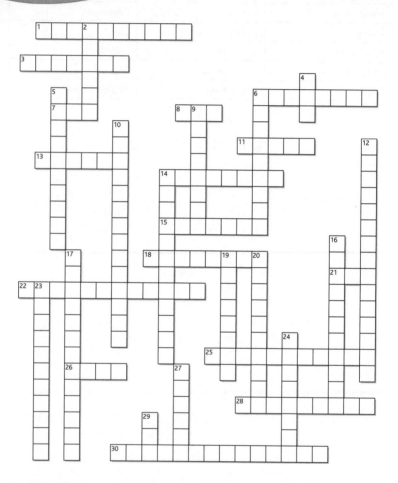

*Meredith Gilliam was a fourth-year medical student at the University of North Carolina at Chapel Hill at the time of this contribution.

Across:

1 - An alpha-1 antagonist used in the treatment of benign prostatic hypertrophy

3 - Most likely diagnosis in an elderly person presenting with a pathologic fracture and "punched-out" lytic bone lesions on plain films: Multiple _____

6 - Term that describes acute onset waxing and waning level of consciousness in your elderly patient

7 - Laboratory value (acronym) classically elevated in elderly woman with unilateral headache and vision loss

8 - Osteitis deformans (Paget disease), which is more common in older adults, is characterized by normal calcium, phosphate, and PTH, but increased _____ (acronym)

11 - To confirm the diagnosis in #20 down, you collect sputum and _____ for testing

13 - Age-related macular degeneration is most likely to present with vision loss in this part of the visual field

14 - An elderly patient who fell 2 weeks ago and has progressive confusion might have this finding on a CT of his head: _____ hematoma

15 - Senile plaques seen on brain microscopy in Alzheimer disease comprises this type of protein

18 - Parkinson disease is associated with this type of rigidity in the arms

21 - The diagnosis suggested by progressive dementia, ataxia, and urinary incontinence in an elderly woman (acronym)

22 - The underlying diagnosis you should suspect in a thin elderly woman presenting with loss of height and kyphosis

25 - An elderly woman with advanced dementia lacks decision-making capacity. Her physician, acting in the patient's best interest, decides to admit her to a skilled nursing facility. What is the ethical principle guiding this physician's action?

26 - Presbycusis causes loss of _____ frequency sounds first

28 - This type of skin carcinoma, common in the elderly, is characterized by rolled edges with central ulceration (two words)

30 - This common condition in older adults is associated with low-fiber diets and increased intraluminal pressure in the distal colon

Down:

2 - Age-related changes may lead to (faster/slower) clearance of fat-soluble drugs

4 - Unlike rheumatoid arthritis, osteoarthritis may affect the _____ joints in the hands (acronym)

5 - This condition may present in elderly patients as "pseudodementia"

6 - Unlike depression, aging is associated with (increased/decreased) REM sleep

9 - Most likely type of dementia in an elderly patient with rigidity, tremor, and hallucinations (two words)

10 - This cardiac valve problem, prevalent in 2% to 9% of adults over 65, causes weak and late peripheral pulses (two words)

12 - This class of drugs is a common first-line treatment for osteoporosis

14 - Keratin pearls on the histopathology of a skin lesion in an older adult suggests this type of carcinoma (two words)

16 - The most common cause of meningitis in the 60+ age group (shorten the genus to an initial)

17 - Synthesis of this neurotransmitter may be reduced in Alzheimer disease

19 - Age-related deficiency of this hormone is the cause of atrophic vaginitis

20 - The organism on the top of your differential when a tour group of octogenarians visiting a whirlpool spa, all get pneumonia (genus)

23 - The most common cause of community-acquired pneumonia in the elderly (shorten the genus to an initial)

24 - To avoid life-threatening hypotension, ask your elderly male patients if they are taking this class of medication before prescribing treatment for erectile dysfunction

27 - After heart disease, the second leading cause of death in adults >65 years old

29 - Vaccination against this virus in >60 years of age group decreases the likelihood of a painful rash (acronym)

Solutions on page 137.

19 Name that Drug!

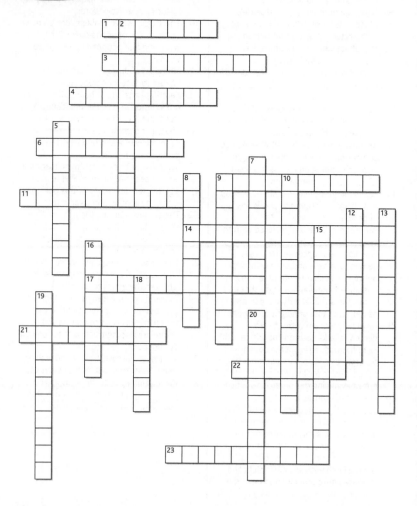

Across:

1 - Nonselectively and irreversibly inhibits cyclooxygenase
3 - Inhibits gastric parietal cell H^+K^+ ATPase
4 - Binds to GABA receptors
6 - Nondihydropyridine blocker of calcium channels
9 - Inhibits loop of Henle sodium and chloride resorption
11 - Nonselectively antagonizes beta-1 and beta-2 adrenergic receptors
14 - Stimulates dopamine receptors
17 - Used in migraine, this activates vascular serotonin 5-HT1 receptors
21 - Relaxes airways by selectively stimulating beta-2 adrenergic receptors
22 - Inhibits sodium–potassium ATPase
23 - Selectively antagonizes H2 receptors

Down:

2 - Inhibits 3-hydroxy-3-methylglutaryl-coenzyme A reductase
5 - Decreases hepatic glucose production, increases insulin sensitivity
7 - Inhibits mast cell degranulation
8 - Stimulates pancreatic islet beta cell insulin release
9 - Selectively inhibits serotonin reuptake
10 - Antagonizes distal convoluted tubule aldosterone receptors
12 - Amide local anesthetic that inhibits Na ion channels
13 - Chelates iron
15 - Reversibly binds and inactivates acetylcholinesterase
16 - Selectively antagonizes angiotensin II AT1 receptors
18 - Antagonizes acetylcholine receptors
19 - Inhibits xanthine oxidase
20 - Inhibits angiotensin-converting enzyme

20 Axis II

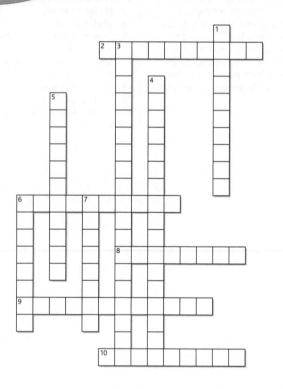

Across:

2 - Cluster B: Unstable, impulsive, vulnerable to abandonment, splitter
6 - Cluster B: Cannot conform to societal rules; criminal behavior
8 - Cluster A: Mistrustful, hostile, suspicious, conspiracy theorist
9 - Cluster B: Grandiose, overly sensitive to criticism, shows little empathy
10 - Cluster C: Insecure, uncomfortable with decision-making or authority

Down:

1 - Cluster B: Overemotional and dramatic
3 - Cluster C: The stubborn perfectionist who likes all the soup cans lined up perfectly (two words)
4 - Cluster C: Noncompliant, procrastinator (two words)
5 - Cluster A: Odd behaviors and thoughts but no psychosis
6 - Cluster C: Involuntarily withdrawn and shy because fears rejection
7 - Cluster A: Purposefully socially withdrawn, content living alone with no friends

Solutions on page 141.

21 Kidney Klues

Yemeng Lu*

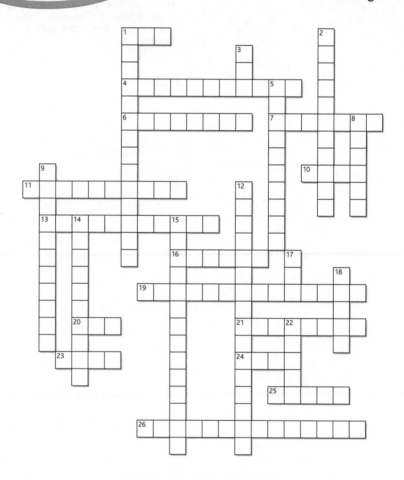

*Yemeng Lu was a third-year medical student at the University of North Carolina at Chapel Hill at the time of this contribution.

Across:

1 - _____ acts on the kidney to decrease renal phosphate reabsorption (acronym)

4 - "S" in MUDPILES for causes of increased anion gap

6 - pH abnormality that leads to hyperkalemia

7 - Manifestation of deficiency of niacin/B3 can resemble _____ disease

10 - A patient loves to eat red meat, fatty seafood, and malt whiskey; he gets a kidney stone that is not visible on x-ray; he most likely also has _____

11 - _____ is moderately secreted by the renal tubules; therefore, it overestimates GFR

13 - A key feature of nephrotic syndrome

16 - Patient with bilateral hearing loss and microscopic hematuria may have _____ syndrome

19 - Your 65-year-old male patient takes 10 minutes to urinate, has a stop-and-go urine stream and still dribbles urine all day; progression of his condition can lead to _____ of the kidneys

20 - _____ nephropathy is the most common lesion found to cause primary glomerulonephritis throughout most developed countries

21 - Early distal convoluted tubule is the site of action for these diuretics

23 - Most common renal malignancy in young children: _____'s tumor

24 - Class of drugs that inhibits the $Na^+/2Cl^-/K^+$ symporters in the thick ascending limb of the nephron: _____ diuretics

25 - A 6-year-old 2 weeks after a strep throat infection with acute poststreptococcal glomerulonephritis will most likely present with _____

26 - Diuretic that can also be used for unfortunate ladies with excess body hair and do not enjoy a 5-o' clock shadow

Down:

1 - A woman with severe dysmenorrhea taking OTC pain medicines ends up with acute renal failure because of the inhibition of production of _____

2 - In the collecting tubules, this leads to insertion of Na^+ channel on the luminal side of the tubule

3 - Consists of modified smooth muscle cells and Na^+ sensing cells (acronym)

5 - A patient with heart failure needs immediate medical diuresis but has a sulfa allergy; you use _____ acid and save the day

8 - "Water under the bridge" = _____ passes under the uterine artery

9 - A potassium-sparing diuretic

12 - Compensatory response to metabolic acidosis

14 - Angiotensin II receptor blockers are less associated with cough compared to ACE inhibitors because they do not increase _____

15 - Patient's leg was crushed in a high-speed MVA and later developed acute tubular necrosis; the mechanism is _____

17 - Inulin is neither secreted nor reabsorbed, thus can be used to approximate _____ (acronym)

18 - Hyponatremia, hypoosmolality, high urine osmolality, and high urine sodium concentration point to _____ (acronym)

22 - CT scan of the patient reveals massively enlarged kidneys bilaterally; he has _____ (acronym)

22 Clinical Scramble

CAREYONDS

HARS

LIPSANES

HACCREN

SHOPTIRECE

DIAGNOSIS: _____

Notes

23 A Gravid Situation

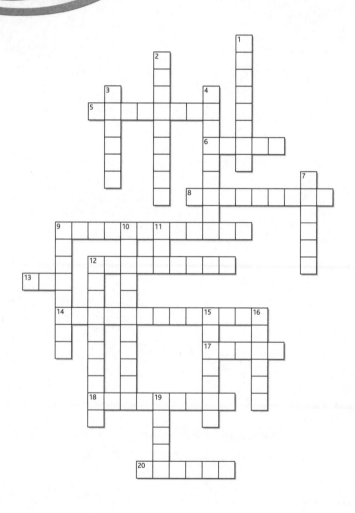

Across:

5 - Nerve block that can ease the pain of childbirth
6 - Stage of labor during which placenta is passed
8 - The "H" in HELLP
9 - Hypertension and proteinuria during the second half of pregnancy
12 - Premature separation of placenta from uterine wall: Placental _____
13 - Elevated in urine and blood if pregnant: Beta-_____ (acronym)
14 - Aspiration of fluid from the amniotic sac for purposes of analysis
17 - Classic acronym for infections that cause birth defects (hint: Not the Olympic one)
18 - #9 across with seizures
20 - Placenta blocking the cervix: Placenta _____

Down:

1 - Hormone that stimulates contractions
2 - Intravenous treatment for preeclampsia while waiting for delivery
3 - Produces progesterone and estrogen during the first trimester: Corpus _____
4 - The "P" in HELLP
7 - Can be performed earlier than #14 across, if needed, to evaluate for genetic abnormalities: Chorionic _____ sampling
9 - Clinically, assume all women of childbearing age are this until you have evidence to the contrary
10 - Most common cause of miscarriage: _____ abnormalities
11 - One of the substances measured to screen for neural tube defects (acronym)
12 - Absence of menses
15 - Implantation outside the uterine cavity: _____ pregnancy
16 - Stage of labor from complete dilation until birth (the "pushing" stage)
19 - "Snowstorm" on ultrasound; cluster of grapes on pathology specimen: _____ pregnancy

Solutions on page 147.

24 Doc, There's a Worm in My...

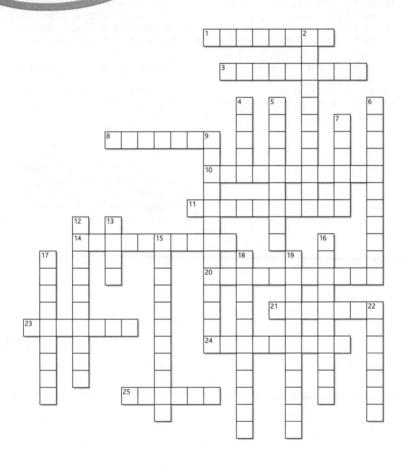

Across:

1 - Beef tapeworm species
3 - Schistosoma species whose egg has a lateral spine
8 - Scotch tape test used to diagnose this infection (common name)
10 - Eating undercooked meat may lead to infection with this (genus), which has the double-barreled egg
11 - Pregnant women should not clean the kitty litter because of possibility of infection with this (genus)
14 - Kala-azar is the visceral form of the infection caused by this genus
20 - Causes cutaneous larvae migrans (genus)
21 - Flagellated protozoan that causes diarrhea (genus)
23 - *Schistosoma haematobium* might infect this if you are peeing in a river in Egypt
24 - Can cause liver abscess: _____ histolytica
25 - Pork tapeworm species

Down:

2 - Causes vaginitis/cervicitis with "strawberry cervix" (genus)
4 - Chagas disease is caused by trypanosoma _____ (species)
5 - Kind of female mosquito that transmits malaria
6 - Causes sleeping sickness: _____ brucei
7 - Double-sounding eye worm disease
9 - Treatment for #2 down
12 - Malaria genus
13 - *Diphyllobothrium latum* is the _____ tapeworm
15 - Antiparasitic used for many worm infections
16 - Pinworm (genus)
17 - "Brain-eating ameba" from warm freshwater up the nose (genus)
18 - Blood fluke (genus)
19 - These kinds of white blood cells are often elevated in parasitic infection
22 - These roundworms can cause an intestinal blockage (genus)

Solutions on page 149.

25 Catching My Breath

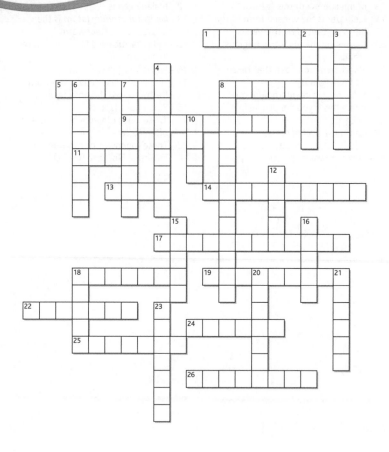

Across:

1 - #7 down + ERV = _____ residual capacity

5 - After you take a normal breath in, the extra volume you can breathe in: Inspiratory _____ volume

8 - Carbon _____ has about 200 times the affinity for hemoglobin than O_2

9 - Type II pneumocytes produce this important stuff

11 - Part of the respiratory tree where no gas exchange takes place: The _____ space

13 - This portion of the lung has some wasted perfusion

14 - The change in lung volume for a given change in pressure

17 - No doubt, one of your favorite things: The oxygen–hemoglobin _____ curve

18 - Bifurcation of this occurs at around T5

19 - C3, C4, and C5 keep this alive

22 - If the lung bud does not completely separate from the esophagus, a tracheoesophageal _____ forms

24 - "A summary of medicine: Air goes in and out, blood goes round and round, and _____ is good"

25 - The left lung has no middle lobe but has this

26 - #5 across + #15 down = inspiratory _____

Down:

2 - Separates right middle lobe from right inferior lobe: _____ fissure

3 - Most of these air sacs actually do not develop until after we are born

4 - When #17 across shifts to the right, there is (increased/decreased) affinity for O_2

6 - The lining of the respiratory tract is derived from this embryonic layer

7 - Volume that stays in the lungs after maximal expiration

8 - Oxidized form of hemoglobin

10 - This portion of the lung has some wasted ventilation

12 - Nonciliated cells with secretory granules: _____ cells

15 - The volume expired with a normal breath: _____ volume

16 - #5 across + #15 down + ERV = _____ capacity

18 - #5 across + #15 down + #7 down + ERV = _____ lung capacity

20 - Provides the electrical "juice" to the diaphragm: _____ nerve

21 - _____ ventilation = TV × respiratory rate

23 - This form of hemoglobin is really ready to bind some O_2

Solutions on page 151.

26 Just for Fun: I'm not a Doctor...*

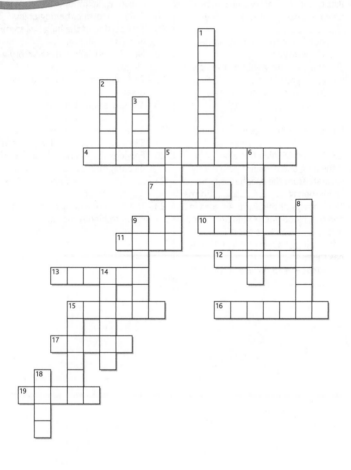

*... but I play one on TV

Across:

4 - Dr. McDreamy's real (well, still fake) name (first and last)
7 - Dr. _____: Medicine Woman
10 - Psychiatrist frequently seen at the bar in Cheers: Dr. _____ Crane
11 - Narcissistic plastic surgeon on Nip/Tuck: Dr. Christian _____
12 - Dr. Kim Briggs, Dr. Molly Clock, Dr. Walter Mickhead, Dr. Grace Miller: Some characters on _____
13 - The Fugitive (was also a movie): Dr. Richard _____
15 - Got his start acting as a doctor on St. Elsewhere: _____ Washington
16 - House's first name (in the show)
17 - Nickname of Dr. Leonard McCoy on the original Star Trek
19 - Little House on the Prairie's doc: Dr. _____

Down:

1 - Dr. Heathcliff _____ in the Cosby Show
2 - Dr. _____ Stevens (nickname) played by Katherine Heigl
3 - Played Carter on ER: Noah _____
5 - One of the two investigators on the X-Files: Dr. Dana _____
6 - Dr. Joel Fleischman: Northern _____
8 - STNG (for the non-Trekkies, that's Star Trek: The Next Generation) doctor Beverly _____
9 - Anthony Edwards' character on ER: Dr. Mark _____
14 - Turned into the Incredible Hulk: Dr. David _____
15 - _____ Howser, MD
18 - Matthew Fox played Dr. _____ Shephard on Lost

27 Codons on Coffee Break

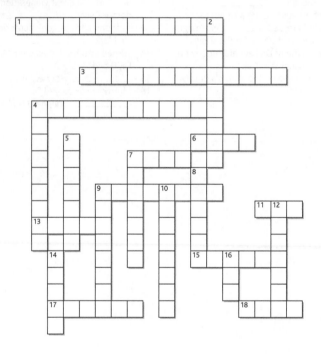

Across:

1 - Deficiency of #2 down causes this type of anemia
3 - An essential amino acid; this one is found in many diet sodas
4 - Cellular site of oxidative phosphorylation (plural)
6 - Element essential for the function of multitude of enzymes. Some say it helps the common cold
7 - A second messenger increased by the activation of a type of G protein
9 - This RNA reads the code
11 - STOP! In the name of this codon (not UAA or UAG)
13 - Laboratory technique in which antigen–antibody reactivity is tested (acronym)
15 - Pellagra is caused by the deficiency of this B vitamin
17 - This genetic structure regulates transcription
18 - The fat-soluble vitamins (alphabetical order)

Down:

2 - Fancier name for vitamin B12
4 - The longest type of RNA
5 - This hormone can be thought of as our storage stimulator
7 - This toxin directly blocks electron flow through the electron transport chain
8 - Muscle cells can be immunochemically stained using this protein
9 - RNA that carries amino acids
10 - Genetic site at which negative regulators bind (also might be seen being used in a different capacity in mafia movies)
12 - One of the purines (would not "The Purines" be a great band name?)
14 - p53 is a _____ suppressor protein
16 - "Let's Get it Started (in Here)" by the Black Eyed Peas might be this codon's theme song

28 Achy Breaky Heart

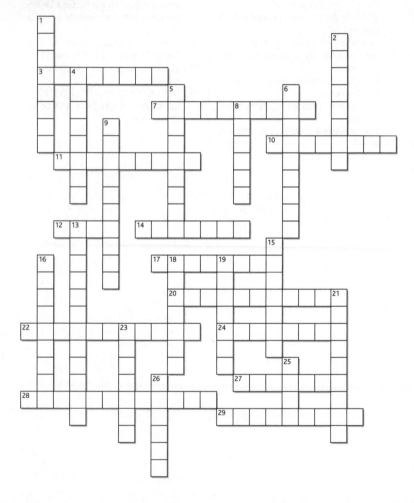

Across:

3 - Cardiac chest pain at rest or escalating in severity = _____ angina

7 - Coronary vasospasm = _____ angina

10 - Vasospasm in the fingers and toes in response to cold temperature or stress

11 - The worrisome sequela of #2 down

12 - Most common cause of right heart failure: _____ heart failure

14 - _____ on exertion is a cardinal symptom of congestive heart failure

17 - Coronary artery aneurysms may be seen as a complication of this syndrome that affects young children: _____ disease

20 - Antineutrophil _____ antibody

22 - Absent femoral pulses on examination, hypertension (in arms), and rib notching: _____ of the aorta

24 - Q waves on ECG in leads II, III, and aVF suggest a prior MI along the _____ wall

27 - Most common site for an aortic aneurysm

28 - Diffuse, upwardly concave ST segment elevation on ECG: Acute _____

29 - Anitschkow cells, previous strep throat, mitral valve stenosis: _____ fever

Down:

1 - This congenital heart defect is associated with aortic stenosis: _____ aortic valve

2 - Elderly woman with unilateral headache and jaw pain might also have stiffness in shoulders: _____ arteritis

4 - Ascending aortic aneurysm may be a result of this infection

5 - Autoimmune pericarditis that can follow a myocardial infarction: _____ syndrome

6 - "Pulseless disease": _____ arteritis

8 - Most common primary cardiac neoplasm in adults: Atrial _____

9 - Heart's response to chronic hypertension = _____ hypertrophy of the left ventricle

13 - Splinter hemorrhages, on examination, in patient with fever: Think _____

15 - Most common type of cardiomyopathy

16 - Cause of isolated right heart failure: Cor _____

18 - Foci of collagen surrounded by lymphocytes and macrophages pathognomonic for rheumatic heart disease: _____ bodies

19 - Thromboangiitis obliterans (Buerger disease) is due to _____

21 - If a patient has stenosis of a right-sided heart valve, consider this syndrome

23 - Antiplatelet drug used for primary and secondary prevention of coronary artery disease

25 - Macrophages ingest oxidized LDL in the vessel wall to become _____ cells

26 - Most frequently infected heart valve

29 It's Raining MEN (and other Endocrine Pathologies)

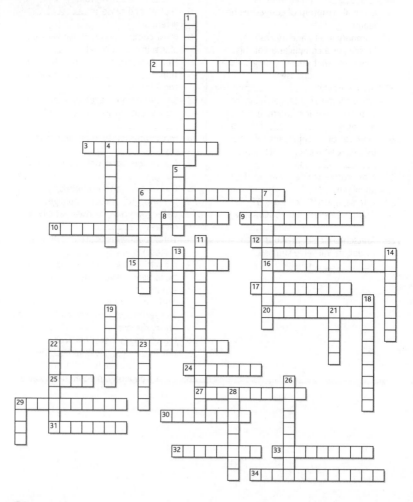

Across:

2 - Name the disease: Weight gain, constipation, dry skin, cold intolerance

3 - Involuntary twitching of facial muscles, when facial nerve is tapped, occurs with this electrolyte abnormality

6 - Checking for these in the urine will clinch the diagnosis of pheochromocytoma

8 - It's Raining MEN: Medullary thyroid cancer, pheochromocytoma, hyperparathyroidism

9 - Antithyroid drug preferred in absence of pregnancy

10 - _____ thyroiditis: A transient hyperthyroid state, associated with a painful goiter, granulomatous inflammation of the thyroid

12 - Pheochromocytoma rule of 10s

15 - _____ thyroiditis: Most common cause of hypothyroidism in adults (eponym)

16 - Drug used in the treatment of central diabetes insipidus

17 - Form of hyperparathyroidism associated with the chronic renal disease, hypocalcemia

20 - Worst thyroid carcinoma

22 - Name the tumor: Paroxysmal hypertension, headache, hyperhidrosis, hyperthermia, hypermetabolism

24 - Form of hyperparathyroidism associated with excess PTH and hypercalcemia

25 - It's Raining MEN: Parathyroid hyperplasia, pancreatic islet cell tumors, pituitary tumors

27 - Medullary thyroid cancer secretes this hormone

29 - These cells migrate from the neural crest and form adrenal medulla

30 - Pheochromocytoma rule of 10s

31 - Name the disease: Hypotension, hyponatremia, hyperpigmentation

32 - Fourth pharyngeal pouch forms the superior/inferior parathyroid

33 - Common cause of mental retardation in the developing world

34 - Name the tumor: Amenorrhea, galactorrhea

Down:

1 - Name the tumor: Malignant abdominal mass in children, related to the N-myc oncogene

4 - Most common thyroid cancer, best prognosis

5 - Name the disease: Tachycardia, exophthalmos, weight loss

6 - Pheochromocytoma rule of 10s

7 - Pheochromocytoma rule of 10s

11 - Antithyroid drug preferred for treating hyperthyroidism in pregnancy

13 - The Rathke's pouch forms the anterior lobe of this gland

14 - Third pharyngeal pouch forms the superior/inferior parathyroid

18 - Name the disease: Large hands and feet

19 - Name the syndrome: Central obesity, moon facies, buffalo hump, abdominal striae

21 - Common cause of hyponatremia, seen in many diseases, classically small-cell lung cancer (acronym)

22 - Histologic "body" may be seen in #4 down and a number of other cancers

23 - It's Raining MEN: Mucosal neuroma, medullary thyroid cancer, marfanoid, pheochromocytoma

26 - Pheochromocytoma rule of 10s

28 - Levels of this byproduct of endogenous insulin production will be low in type I diabetes and high in type II diabetes

29 - Name the syndrome: Hypertension, hypokalemia, low renin level

Solutions on page 159.

30 A Bug's Life 2

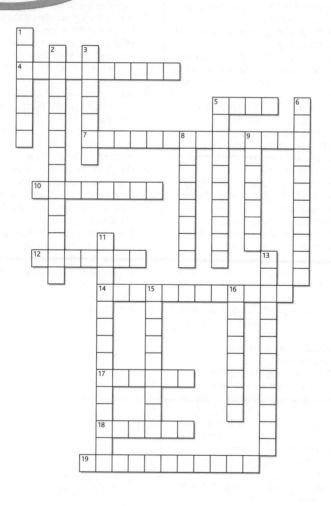

Across:

4 - Group B strep is also known as streptococcus _____ (species)

5 - Group A strep are _____
-hemolytic

7 - Catalase-positive, gram-positive cocci
(genus)

10 - A spore-forming, gram-positive rod
genus (think bad fried rice)

12 – You will find most DNA viruses replicating here

14 - Gram-positive cocci in chains (genus)

17 - They have no DNA or RNA, but can
still cause an infection

18 - Use this smear of a sample from an
unroofed vesicle to test for herpes

19 - This lactose nonfermenting gram-
negative rod is oxidase-positive
(genus only)

Down:

1 - Primary syphilis presents with a
painless _____

2 - Double-stranded circular DNA virus
that causes warts

3 - *Neisseria meningitidis* ferments this
sugar

5 - Group A strep are _____
-sensitive (and this drug can be used
topically for impetigo)

6 - A board question about cat bites
should make you think of this organism (genus)

8 - The only gram-positive with lipopolysaccharide-lipid A (genus)

9 - The toxin from it causes severe
watery diarrhea by overactivating
adenylate cyclase

11 - The organism that causes plague (two
words)

13 - Gram-positive and acid-fast (genus,
plural)

15 - Gram-negatives often contain this
heat-stable lipopolysaccharide in
their outer membrane (it makes
people sick)

16 - *S. pneumoniae* and *S. viridans*,
both alpha-hemolytic, can be told
apart because *S. pneumoniae* is
_____ sensitive

Solutions on page 161.

31 Inheritance

```
V E G A R O T S N E G O C Y L G D U N E C G
X L G P Y B O S P H E R O C Y T O S I S V I
R Q N A F R A M H M U E D G Y G Y S O S I Z
B M Q J P F L E J F A M D F Z X H S I G P N
P Y U C O L Q O I H O C Z U C I S S F T H L
J S O G Y S D P M X L V C H H I O X B T R N
N Z X Z R I D K G L E U Q G S R B A O M A D
E Q N Q N C Q L W F C D M O E A I S F Z N K
U J F R D K G E X Q Z M T L T R A I R I T B
R H Q W J L M Z R Q S A C V U A E S J I I S
O D W T Y E L W S I M S U N O I J O G J T V
F R U I T C O R N O S J O W N M V R P B R G
I S H Z N E Y I R U T T G V A E C B Z F Y P
B Z D F Z L B H O A E C L G Q S E I L B P M
R Z N P O L C R X K A E F X P S W F F R S S
O S D Q A O E O L H O M U B U A O C Z P I N
M U P C M B S Y U Y U G Q Z L L Z I O L N H
A Z B E U D N F C F M N K V M A L T T Y D W
T J H T J E M P H A E L T E W H T S A D E Y
O J I G H W I S H A P J I I D T H Y I M F E
S I C P A I C L A F S M D H N O A C P F I M
I V O S C H E U E V D X Q J W G E U J U C C
S H H Q C P U N J J T Z Y L B W T W T F I V
Y E J A S F U R Z N Q L C T R Y J O N Z E G
H U A D N I L L E P P I H N O V L Y N J N O
E W U C Q S K A S H K V R S Q E M E V E C S
X Z T I C C H S Z F R X L G X U I V L L Y H
J G S E L E R K S D O R P E W J X J J W N O
```

Albinism	Antitrypsin deficiency	Cystic fibrosis
Glycogen storage	Hemochromatosis	Huntington
Marfan	Neurofibromatosis	Phenylketonuria
Sickle cell	Spherocytosis	Thalassemia
Tuberous sclerosis	Von Hippel–Lindau	

Solutions on page 162.

32 My Neurotransmitters are Acting Up

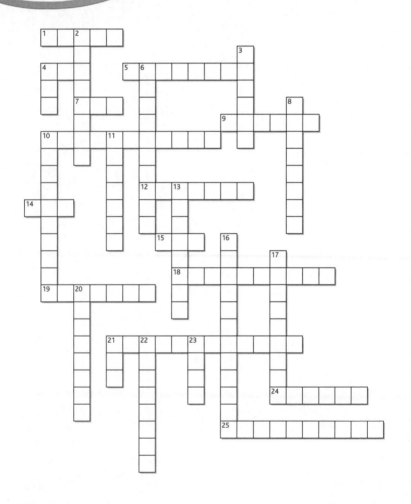

Across:

1 - Rarely seen paralysis from damage to LMNs caused by this virus
4 - Most common cause of neonatal meningitis (acronym)
5 - Degeneration of mamillary bodies results from deficiency of this vitamin
7 - Location of the ring seen in #9 across
9 - Liver disease which causes copper accumulation
10 - Most common neural tube defect (two words)
12 - Neurotoxin that inhibits glycine release
14 - This trinucleotide repeat leads sufferers to "dance"
15 - Xanthochromia and RBCs in the CSF should raise suspicion for this infection (acronym)
18 - Part of the brain most sensitive to alcohol
19 - Seizure of childhood characterized by blank stare
21 - This metabolic abnormality may create a stroke mimic
24 - Negri bodies are seen in this uniformly fatal disease
25 - Neurotoxin that blocks glycine receptor

Down:

2 - Bug that causes meningitis only in the very young or very old
3 - Arnold–Chiari malformation leads to herniation of this cerebellar structure
4 - Pseudopalisading arrangement of cells characterizes this devastating CNS tumor (acronym)
6 - Disease of #14 across
8 - Depletion of this neurotransmitter leads to a disorder characterized by a resting tremor
10 - Tumor often seen bilaterally in neurofibromatosis type 2
11 - Guillain–Barre syndrome is a post-viral ascending paralysis with high _____ levels in the CSF
13 - Deficiency in hexosaminidase A, cherry-red spot on macula
16 - Most common cause of meningitis in elderly (species form)
17 - This most common form of dementia occurs at earlier age in individuals with trisomy 21
20 - Loss of touch, vibration, proprioception to the lower extremities caused by advanced form of this infection
21 - Cause of meningitis in children on the decline, thanks to this immunization (acronym)
22 - Histologic features of meningioma: _____ body (also seen in a variety of other tumors)
23 - Type of "body" seen histologically in #8 down

Solutions on page 165.

33 GI Fizziology

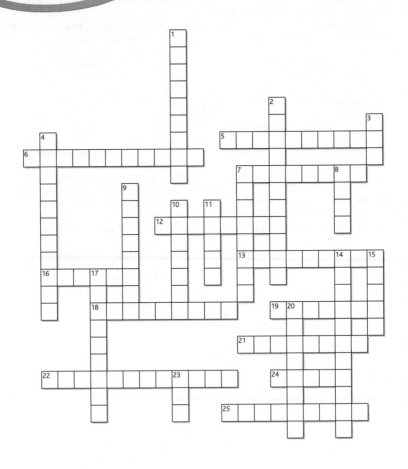

Across:

5 - Direct bilirubin is conjugated with this acid before being excreted in bile

6 - CCK stimulates contraction of this (Useless hint: Not the uterus)

7 - These cells secrete gastric acid

12 - Hormone that acts on the pancreatic ductal cells to increase mucus and bicarb secretion

13 - Binds vitamin B12 for absorption in terminal ileum: _____ factor

16 - Your pancreas probably secretes a lot of this after you eat at your favorite fast food restaurant

18 - Mast cells secrete this

19 - Secreted by salivary glands, this helps digest starches

21 - Lipase turns triglycerides into fatty acids and this

22 - The D cells secrete this

24 - If your patient has a tumor that is producing a lot of gastrin, a potential complication is this

25 - If histamine is blocked, gastric acid (increases/decreases)

Down:

1 - If prostaglandin production is decreased, gastric acid (increases/decreases)

2 - The presence of this in the stomach helps neutralize the acid

3 - The I cells of the duodenum and jejunum secrete this (acronym)

4 - My mom always says food goes "right through her"; what she does not understand is this reflex

7 - Pepsinogen comes in handy to digest these

8 - Acetylcholine stimulates production of this in the stomach

9 - CCK also stimulates the acinar cells of the pancreas to release these (Hint: The first letter is worth 10 points in Scrabble)

10 - Folate is absorbed in this part of the intestine

11 - Small intestine "border" that when wiped out can lead to diarrhea

14 - If your intestines are not absorbing fat properly (say, because your ileum is missing), you might develop "greasy stools"; this is called

_____

15 - These cells secrete pepsinogen

17 - Enzyme that turns CO_2 and H_2O into H^+ and HCO_3^-: Carbonic

_____

20 - Long-chain fatty acids form these prior to passive diffusion

23 - The stomach's proton pump is an H^+/K^+ _____ ase pump

Solutions on page 167.

34 BMJ (Bones, Muscles, Joints)

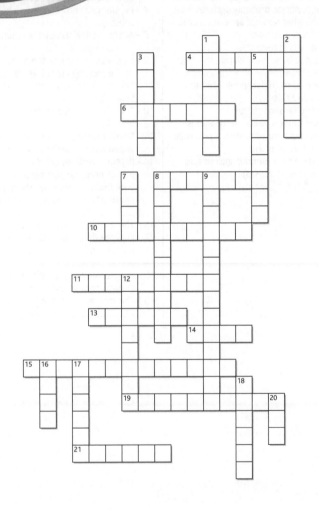

Across:

4 - Released from sarcoplasmic reticulum in response to #9 down

6 - Disease of poor calcification of bone leading to bowing of legs in children

8 - If you were one of these kinds of muscle fibers your disks would be intercalated

10 - Pannus formation in joints = _____ arthritis

11 - Legg–Calve–Perthes disease is _____ necrosis of the head of the femur

13 - Actin and _____ interact to generate a muscle contraction

14 - Lifting weights results in hypertrophy of _____ twitch muscle fibers

15 - Hereditary disorder of defective osteoclasts leading to bone over-growth

19 - Your patient with sickle cell has osteomyelitis, so be sure to consider this bug (genus)

21 - If you have bad proline and lysine hydroxylation, you may be suffering from _____

Down:

1 - Slipped _____ femoral epiphysis

2 - Gap junctions are present in this type of muscle fibers

3 - Osgood–Schlatter disease is knee pain in an active teenager resulting from partial avulsion of this tuberosity

5 - Blue sclerae: Osteogenesis _____

7 - Tick-borne disease that can cause arthritis

8 - Calcium binds to _____ to activate myosin light-chain kinase

9 - To start the process of skeletal muscle contraction, action potentials cause _____ of T-tubules

12 - Dry eyes, dry mouth, arthritis just might be this syndrome

16 - Type 1 muscle fibers are _____ twitch

17 - "Onion skin" appearance in bones: _____ sarcoma

18 - Sarcomere separators

20 - Binds to myosin head and releases actin (acronym)

Solutions on page 169.

35 Your Nephrolithiasis Test Came Back...*

Yemeng Lu**

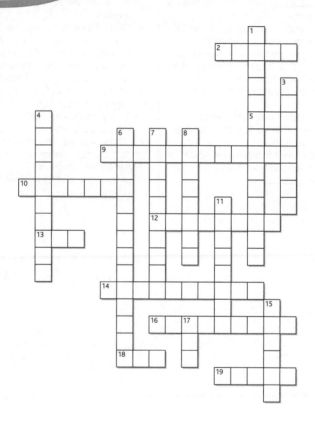

*...unfortunately, you didn't pass.

**Yemeng Lu was a third-year medical student at the University of North Carolina at Chapel Hill at the time of this contribution.

Across:

2 - Histologic examination of a mass shows embryonic glomerular structures in a spindle-cell stroma in a patient with chromosome 11 mutations; this suggests _____ tumor

5 - Linear deposits of _____ along the basement membrane = Goodpasture syndrome

9 - Renal biopsy shows reduplication of the elastic lamina and fibrosis of the media of the arcuate arteries; the patient most likely has _____

10 - _____ change disease on electron microscopy shows podocyte effacement

12 - "A" in WAGR complex stands for _____

13 - Overgrowth of renal polygonal clear cells filled with lipids and carbohydrates lead to (acronym)

14 - Goodpasture syndrome, Wegener's granulomatosis, and microscopic polyangiitis can all result in _____ glomerulonephritis

16 - The visceral layer of the Bowman's capsule is consistent of these cells

18 - Patient with skin rash and bilateral arthritis of the knee also has RBC casts on urine analysis, most likely has _____ (acronym)

19 - Acute post-_____ (short form) glomerulonephritis has immune complex deposition humps located subepithelially in the glomerulus

Down:

1 - Treatment for cystine kidney stones involves _____ of the urine

3 - Triad of necrotizing granulomas of the upper airways, renal disease, and vasculitis = _____ granulomatosis

4 - An 8-year-old boy with hexagonal crystals in his urine and a positive nitroprusside cyanide test of the urine has _____

6 - Kidney at autopsy shows purulent inflammation and accumulation of pus in the renal pelvis; the patient most likely died from

7 - Type of glomerulonephritis with "spike and dome" appearance on electron microscopy showing subepithelial deposits

8 - A woman with neurogenic bladder presenting with an indwelling catheter is found to have a 3-cm stone filling the renal pelvis, most likely composed of _____

11 - Kimmelstiel–Wilson lesion = _____ nephropathy

15 - A man with a recent upper respiratory tract infection also has microscopic hematuria, most likely has _____ disease

17 - A woman with retained products of conception dies from _____ (acronym) and autopsy shows ischemic necrosis of both kidney cortices

36 Private Parts Path

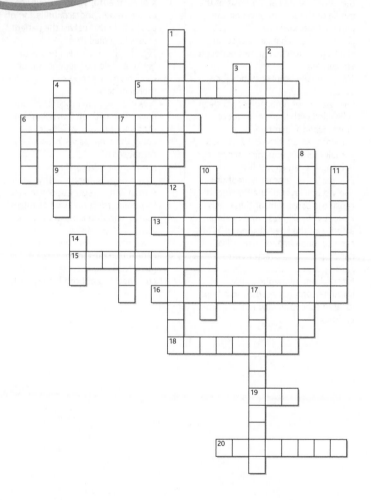

Across:

5 - Dilated veins of the pampiniform plexus, more common on the left

6 - Painful intercourse

9 - Struma ovarii contains tissue that can produce this hormone

13 - Small, mobile, firm breast mass in a young woman that increases in tenderness with menstruation is most likely this benign tumor

15 - Bloody nipple discharge suggests intraductal _____

16 - Men on spironolactone might complain of "growing breasts"; the medical term is _____

18 - Most common testicular tumor

19 - Virus associated with cervical cancer (acronym)

20 - When the Viagra commercial warns of a painful erection lasting more than 4 hours, it is referring to this condition

Down:

1 - Common name for leiomyomata of the uterus

2 - Milky nipple discharge

3 - Amenorrhea (and infertility), hirsutism, obesity: Clues to this (acronym)

4 - Infection of the breast that can lead to abscess

6 - Early breast malignancy that has not invaded basement membrane (acronym)

7 - This cancer is the most common GYN malignancy

8 - This "disease" is a common cause of breast lumps in young women

10 - Prolonged estrogen exposure (increases/decreases) risk of breast cancer

11 - Ovarian germ cell tumor; it is pretty freaky because it may contain teeth and hair

12 - Cells of cervical dysplasia

14 - Common cause of urinary outflow symptoms in older men (acronym)

17 - Abnormally heavy menstrual bleeding

Solutions on page 173.

37 This Puzzle May Take You a Lung Time

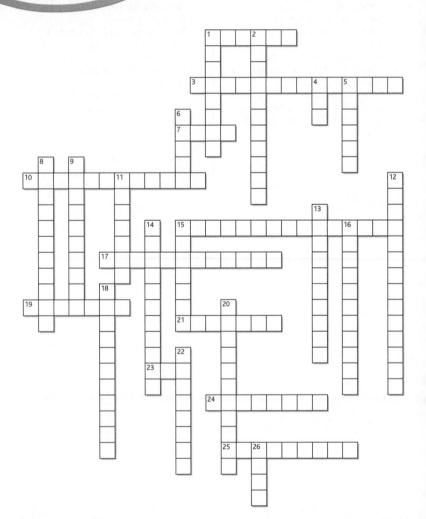

Across:

1 - Clotting triad 1/3: Venous
_____

3 - Recurrent infections in patients with cystic fibrosis may develop this condition of chronically dilated bronchioles

7 - Severe lung injury resulting from a variety of causes, commonly severe infection and systemic inflammatory disorders (acronym)

10 - This may occur spontaneously in tall, thin adolescent and young adult men

15 - Clotting triad 3/3: _____ state

17 - Another pulmonary–renal syndrome; this disease is caused by antibodies to basement membrane

19 - Eponym of clotting triad

21 - This protein is degraded in excess in the disease described in #8 down

23 - Levels of this enzyme may be increased in #2 down (acronym)

24 - Pulmonary _____: Possible cause of sudden death in patients with #19 across

25 - Probably the most widely used inhaled, short-acting beta2-agonist

Down:

1 - This drug class exerts its anti-inflammatory effects via inhibition of leukotriene synthesis

2 - A systemic disease pathologically characterized by the presence of noncaseating granulomas

4 - Fluid-filled alveoli may be the result of this clinical entity (acronym)

5 - Many people carry around metered dose inhalers of the drug in #25 across for its rapid effects in treating attacks of this common disease

6 - Antibody seen in #22 down (acronym)

8 - You might suspect deficiency of the enzyme alpha-1-_____ in a young patient with COPD and liver disease

9 - Ipratropium prevents bronchoconstriction by antagonism of this receptor

11 - If a one-way valve mechanism is present, you may develop a _____ pneumothorax

12 - This finding, on physical examination, is characteristic of #10 across

13 - Deficiency of this molecule leads to the neonatal equivalent of #7 across

14 - Clotting triad 2/3: _____ injury

15 - Formation of these pathologic "membranes" is associated with #7 across and #13 down

16 - Collapsed or unexpanded lung tissue

18 - This drug is a leukotriene receptor antagonist

20 - This bug often chronically colonizes and recurrently infects patients with cystic fibrosis

22 - A rare pulmonary–renal syndrome; the patient may be a young male presenting with bleeding from the upper and lower respiratory tracts and granulomas

26 - Certain types of hypersensitivity pneumonitis may be due to exposure to antigens from this animal

Solutions on page 175.

38 Clinical Scramble

ANEWJAY

NOSESIL

REEVF

DRACCIA

RUMMUR

THOR

STOPS

LORES

SONDE

ANSWER: _____

Notes

39 Bug Killers

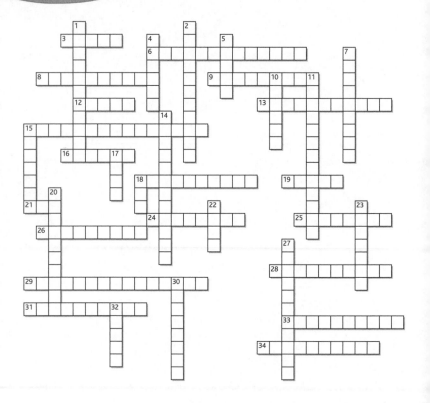

Across:

3 - Use of tetracyclines in childhood may cause discoloration of these

6 - Used for the treatment of anaerobic infections and protozoa

8 - DNA synthesis inhibitors, used for gram-negative infections

9 - This antibiotic must be given with pyridoxine to prevent neurotoxicity

12 - This "terrible" drug works well for fungal infections (short form)

13 - Treatment of choice for most tick-borne illness

15 - Irreversibly bind the 30S ribosome

16 - Quick infusion of vancomycin may result in this syndrome (two words)

18 - Developed for influenza A, but also useful for Parkinson disease

19 - _____ generation cephalosporins: Good gram-negative coverage, weaker gram-positive

21 - Percent of allergic cross-sensitivity between penicillins and cephalosporins

24 - Class that inhibits cell wall synthesis (initial the first word)

25 - Drug used in prophylaxis for contacts of meningococcal cases

26 - Only oral agent with no MRSA resistance

28 - Metronidazole may cause a _____-like reaction when combined with alcohol

29 - Rarely used agent, associated with aplastic anemia and gray baby syndrome

31 - Great gram-negative and Pseudomonas coverage, but nasty effects on hearing and kidneys

33 - Antimalarial known for CNS side effects

34 - Bind the 23S RNA of the 50S ribosome

Down:

1 - Antihelminthic, useful for variety of worm infestations

2 - Class of "biggest guns" cover all bugs except MRSA

4 - Antibiotic associated with Stevens–Johnson syndrome (acronym)

5 - _____ generation cephalosporins: Good gram-positive coverage, weak gram-negative

7 - Guanosine analog, inhibits viral DNA polymerase, useful for herpes viruses

10 - Class of antifungals that inhibit ergosterol synthesis

11 - Oral B-lactam that covers *S. aureus*, but NOT MRSA

14 - Penicillin with Pseudomonas coverage

15 - Frequently used in concert with ceftriaxone to provide "atypical" coverage in pneumonia (First three syllables)

17 - B-lactam with added activity to gram-negative rods: _____ icillin

18 - Antiretroviral drug used to prevent maternal–fetal HIV transmission (acronym)

20 - Still works great for Group A Streptococcus and syphilis

22 - Best bet for MRSA treatment: _____omycin

23 - Amoxicillin, clarithromycin, and metronidazole: A triple therapy for this bug (initial first word)

27 - Covers gram-positive, anaerobes, some MRSA, but high association with *C. difficile* superinfection

30 - Broadest spectrum cephalosporin, covers Pseudomonas as well

32 - Young female with spontaneous Achilles tendon rupture may be on this drug for her UTI (short form)

40 BuzzWards

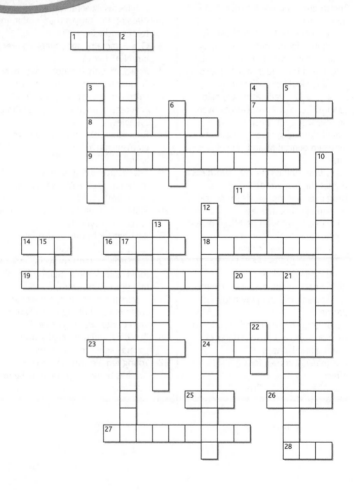

Across:

1 - Slapped cheek
(_____ disease)
7 - Butterfly rash
8 - Starry sky B-cells
9 - Chocolate cyst
11 - Basophilic stippling (toxin)
14 - Auer rods (acronym)
16 - "Bunch of grapes" or "snowstorm"
on ultrasound (_____
pregnancy)
18 - Neoplasm with teeth
19 - Thumb sign
20 - Rocker bottom feet (_____
syndrome)
23 - Exophthalmos
24 - Buffalo hump
25 - Muddy brown casts (acronym)
26 - Bull's eye rash
27 - Flushing and diarrhea
28 - Worst headache of my life (acronym)

Down:

2 - Shield chest
(_____ syndrome)
3 - Coffee ground emesis (acronym)
4 - Currant jelly sputum (bug)
5 - Honeycomb lung (acronym)
6 - Strawberry tongue (bug, short form)
10 - Splinter hemorrhages
12 - Currant jelly stool
13 - Bag of worms
15 - Midsystolic click (acronym)
17 - Sunburst on bone x-ray
21 - Sulfur granules (bug)
22 - Nutmeg liver (underlying cause,
acronym)

Solutions on page 181.

41 Out Damned Spot!*

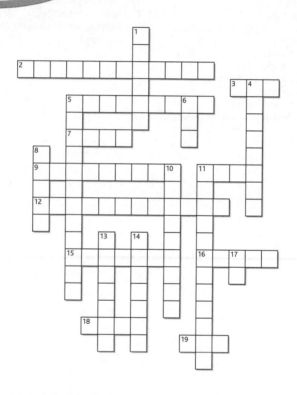

*The spot was an imagined blood stain seen by Lady Macbeth in Shakespeare's Macbeth.

Across:

2 - t(9:22) results in _____ chromosome which results in leukemia

3 - Most common hereditary bleeding disorder (acronym)

5 - ITP is due to antibodies against these

7 - Basophilic stippling seen in _____ toxicity

9 - #12 across count is (increased/decreased) in hemolytic anemia

11 - Rods seen in acute myeloblastic leukemia

12 - Nonnucleated immature RBC formed in bone marrow

15 - Lytic lesions on plain x-ray, think multiple _____

16 - These bodies are seen in G6PD deficiency (hint: Ketchup and 57)

18 - Hemophilia A is the deficiency of factor _____ (Roman numeral)

19 - A severely ill patient with elevated level of fibrin split products, elevated D-dimer, and low level of fibrinogen has this (acronym)

Down:

1 - If you are missing this, you might have Howell–Jolly bodies in your peripheral blood smear

4 - Follow the INR (a reflection of PT) to assess effect of this drug

5 - Increased RBC mass could be _____ vera

6 - Low platelets, anemia, fever, renal failure, and neurologic changes, think this (acronym)

8 - Iron deficiency anemia is _____cytic

10 - Ristocetin aggregation is (increased/decreased) in vWF deficiency

11 - #13 down binds to _____-III

13 - Monitor aPTT to assess the effect of this drug

14 - Reed–Sternberg cells seen in _____ disease

17 - Hemophilia B is the deficiency of factor _____ (Roman numeral)

Solutions on page 183.

42 Doc, I Think It's My Connective Tissue*

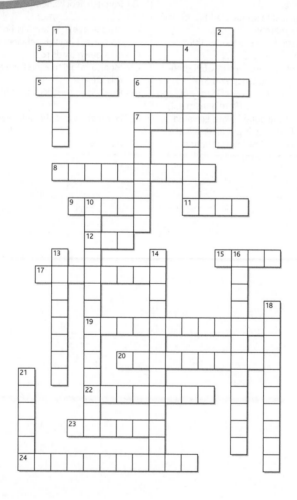

*Probably something a patient will never say.

Across:

3 - One of the DMARDs
5 - Anti-_____ antibodies are highly specific for lupus
6 - A child with bowed legs and thin skull bones probably has _____
7 - One of the 6P's of compartment syndrome
8 - Boutonniere deformity is usually seen in this type of arthritis
9 - Classic rash of lupus
11 - Uric acid crystals in joints
12 - _____B27
15 - TB of the spine: _____ disease
17 - It is the R in CREST syndrome
19 - A primary bone malignancy
20 - Calcium pyrophosphate crystal deposition in joints
22 - A patient with dry eyes, dry mouth, and arthritis may have _____ syndrome
23 - Beethoven, who had a prominent forehead and hearing loss, might have had this disease of abnormal bone activity
24 - Noncaseating granulomatous disease

Down:

1 - Heliotrope rash is classic for _____myositis
2 - Conjunctivitis, urethritis, and arthritis: _____ syndrome
4 - #12 across is associated with _____ spondylitis
7 - Gout of the big toe
10 - Most common cause of dwarfism
13 - Allopurinol, a treatment for gout, inhibits _____ oxidase
14 - "Marble bones"
16 - Condition of decreased bone density
18 - "Sausage fingers"
21 - A type of aggressive sarcoma, mostly affecting young boys

Solutions on page 185.

43 Clues in a Drug's Name

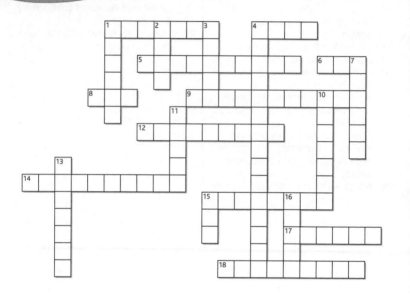

Across:

1 - The "-dipines" are the dihydropyridine form of these channel blockers
4 - If a drug ends in -olol, there is a good chance it blocks these receptors
5 - "-mabs" are _____ antibodies
6 - You will find these three letters in the names of many cephalosporins
8 - If your patient is on a drug ending in -avir, -udine, or both, he probably has this infection (acronym)
9 - Drugs that block this receptor (the type II AT1) end in -sartan
12 - Drugs ending in -etine or -opram block reuptake of this
14 - "-floxacins" are this class of antibiotics
15 - Medications for acute migraine
17 - Drugs that block this pump often end in -prazole
18 - Drugs ending in -tidine, like ranitidine, block these receptors

Down:

1 - Drugs ending in this inhibit mucopeptide synthesis in the bacterial cell wall
2 - If you are calling stat for a drug ending in -plase, you are probably trying to break up one of these somewhere (Useless hint: Not a fight)
3 - Macrolides often end in these five letters
4 - These typically end in -lam or -pam
7 - "-azoles" are anti-_____
10 - HMG-CoA reductase inhibitors
11 - ACE inhibitors
13 - Drugs with this ending help lower triglycerides
15 - A "-triptyline" is one of this class of drugs (acronym)
16 - Drugs ending in -azosin block peripheral _____ receptors

44 What is the Most Common...?

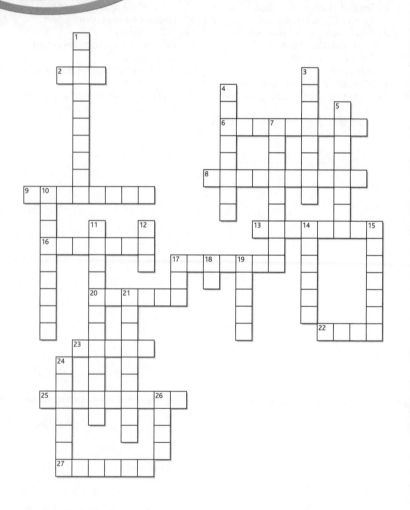

Across:

2 - Congenital heart defect (acronym)
6 - Cause of intestinal obstruction
8 - Cause of dementia
9 - Cancer in men
13 - Cause of chronic kidney disease
16 - Cause of primary hyperparathyroidism
17 - Cause of cirrhosis
20 - Valve affected by rheumatic fever
22 - Cause of cancer death
23 - Chromosomal disorder
   (_____ syndrome)
25 - Cause of death in Alzheimer patients
27 - Cancer of the heart

Down:

1 - Cause of hypothyroidism
3 - Cancer of the testes
4 - Heritable cause of mental retardation
5 - Type of hernia
7 - Form of hypertension
10 - Bug causing diarrhea in children
11 - Bug in community-acquired
   pneumonia
12 - Artery for MI (acronym)
14 - Cancer in women
15 - Preventable cause of death
17 - Cause of leukemia in young children
   (acronym)
18 - Fatal genetic disease in Caucasians
   (acronym)
19 - Cause of death in US (organ)
21 - Cause of congenital adrenal hyperplasia (_____-hydroxylase
   deficiency)
24 - Worm infection in US
26 - Dietary deficiency

Solutions on page 189.

45 This Puzzle Takes Guts

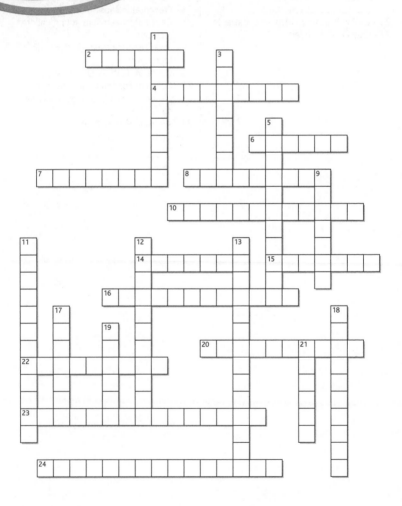

Across:

2 - Kayser–Fleischer rings: _____ disease
4 - "Bird beak" esophagus (on barium swallow)
6 - Pharyngeal pouch in which food can get stuck: _____ diverticulum
7 - Metaplasia in distal esophagus
8 - Trouble swallowing
10 - Hamartomas of GI tract and hyperpigmentation: _____–_____ syndrome
14 - Duodenal ulcers are associated with this germ (only use first initial of genus)
15 - Most common site of colon cancer
16 - If you drink too much after your Step 1 exam, leading to vomiting that tears your esophagus, it is called a _____–_____ tear
20 - Organism responsible for pseudo-membranous colitis (only use first initial of genus)
22 - Antimitochondrial antibodies are seen in primary biliary _____
23 - Telescoping intestines
24 - Two-word diagnosis if you feel an "olive" in the epigastrium of a 2-week-old boy who has been having projectile vomiting

Down:

1 - Most common cause of diarrhea in infants
3 - Twisting intestines
5 - Blood in the vomit
9 - Precancerous colon polyp
11 - Pain at McBurney's point associated with anorexia suggests this diagnosis
12 - #17 down suggests this diagnosis
13 - Common cause of lower GI bleeding
17 - Fever, jaundice, RUQ pain: _____ triad
18 - Major cause of acute pancreatitis
19 - Skip lesions in the colon
21 - Gluten sensitivity: _____ disease

Solutions on page 191.

46 A Biased Puzzle?

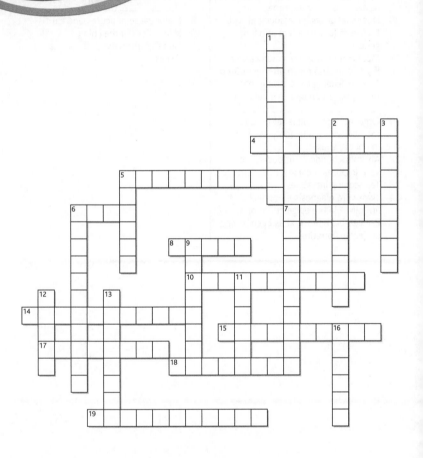

Across:

4 - The proportion of people who develop an outcome over a given time period

5 - A cross-sectional study is sometimes called a _____ study because it can be used to estimate this

6 - A _____-analysis is a kind of study that mathematically pools the data from multiple studies to generate a "best" estimate

7 - Prevalence of a disease in a population of patients can be used as an estimate of the _____ probability

8 - The odds of the outcome among the exposed group divided by the odds of the outcome among the nonexposed group is the odds _____

10 - For a diagnostic test, true negatives divided by true negatives plus false positives

14 - An investigator selects 20 medical students who have Step 1 Exam phobia and 20 students who do not; she then calls them and asks whether they ever did CrossWard puzzles to see if there is an association; this is a _____ study (two words)

15 - The interval that represents the range of values expected 95 out of 100 times (if a study is repeated 100 times) is the 95% _____ interval

17 - A highly _____ test when positive is helpful at ruling in disease

18 - The posttest probability of a disease given a negative test is equal to 1 minus the _____ predictive value

19 - Test X detects 97% of disease among people who have the disease; 97% is the _____

Down:

1 - In a study that shows gray hair is associated with coronary artery disease, age is a _____

2 - For a diagnostic test, true positives divided by true positives plus false negatives

3 - When a lot of people in one group of a study drop out and few in the other group drop out, this is a potential _____ bias

5 - By convention (and quite arbitrarily), a study's finding is considered statistically significant if this is <0.05

6 - A study bias in which it is easier to tell if people in one group had the outcome is a differential _____ bias

7 - For a diagnostic test, true positives divided by all positives: Positive _____ value

9 - Drug A reduces blood clots by 5% while Drug B reduces blood clots by 2.5%; the _____ risk reduction is 2.5%

11 - An investigator identifies 800 people free of syndrome Z and follows them over time to see if exposure to energy drinks is associated with development of syndrome Z; this is a _____ study design

12 - The positive test in a patient with a very low pretest probability is likely to be a _____ positive test

13 - The posttest probability of a disease given a positive test is the _____ predictive value

16 - The inverse of the absolute risk reduction is the _____ needed to treat

Solutions on page 193.

47 Can You "Crack" this Puzzle?

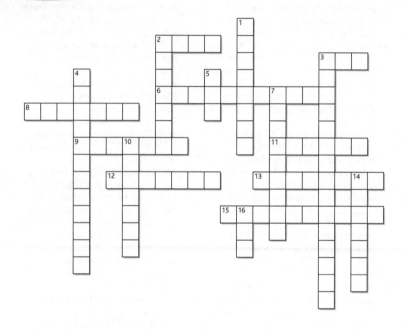

Across:

2 - GHB, ketamine, and roofies are known as "_____ drugs" because of where teenagers use them
3 - Hallucinogen that is a NMDA receptor agonist (acronym)
6 - Causes increased catecholamine release
8 - Gamma-_____-butyric acid
9 - Whippets, poppers, and snappers are all taken by this method
11 - Street name "smack"
12 - MDMA common name
13 - "Roofies"
15 - Used to treat benzodiazepine overdose

Down:

1 - This can stimulate and relax
2 - Blocks norepinephrine, dopamine, and serotonin reuptake
3 - This decongestant is no longer available directly on store shelves because it is an ingredient in meth labs
4 - Potentiate GABA's action by keeping chloride channels open
5 - Active compound in marijuana (acronym)
7 - Psilocybin: Street name "magic _____" (Hint: Not "Mike")
10 - Withdrawal can lead to delirium tremens
14 - Overdose of this class of drugs can cause pinpoint pupils and respiratory depression
16 - Withdrawal leads to flashbacks (acronym)

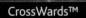

48 Clinical Scramble

VEERF

LOSTKEYOUSIC

CAPETHANY

CINTIFONE

IPENNYSHOOT

ANSWER: _____

Notes

49 This Puzzle is More Fun than a Fungus Ball

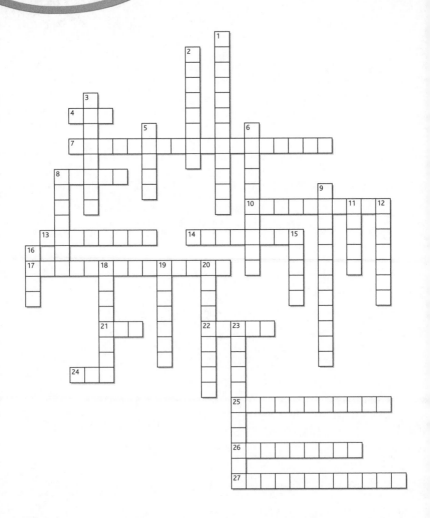

Across:

4 - Deletion of this amino acid, responsible for the most common fatal genetic disease in caucasians (acronym)

7 - Fungal pneumonia seen in the American Southwest

8 - Pott disease: Extrapulmonary form of TB that affects the _____

10 - This atypical pneumonia bug (genus) lives in the water supply and may be associated with outbreaks

13 - _____ ileus: Form of small-bowel obstruction seen in infants, may be a presentation of CF

14 - Exposure to this mineral increases the risk of bronchogenic carcinoma and mesothelioma

17 - Fungal infection common in Ohio and Mississippi River Valleys

21 - This virus causes endless cases of viral pneumonias and bronchiolitis in children during winter months (acronym)

22 - _____ lobe: Usual site of secondary tuberculosis

24 - Most common cause of pneumonia in a newborn (acronym)

25 - Fungal infection which may form a fungus ball

26 - Lung cancer associated with poor prognosis and paraneoplastic syndromes (two words)

27 - Cancer strongly associated with smoking and in central location (also two words)

Down:

1 - The most common bug causing typical pneumonia (species form)

2 - Treatment of active TB with this drug may turn your urine orange

3 - Electrolyte transport affected by #4 across

5 - _____ carcinoma: Most common type of lung cancer

6 - _____ pneumoniae: One of the "atypicals" and the cause of "walking pneumonia"

8 - Secondary infection with this bug may occur in primary infection due to #20 down (initial the genus)

9 - Life-threatening pneumonia in immunocompromised patients, especially HIV

11 - _____ lobe: Usual location of #16 down

12 - Staphylococcal pneumonia may lead to the formation of this cavitary lesion

15 - _____ test: Diagnostic test for CF

16 - _____ complex: Caseating granuloma seen in primary tuberculosis

18 - Other nonlung organ primarily affected in patients with cystic fibrosis

19 - _____ TB: Tuberculosis outside of the lung

20 - Frequent seasonal mutations require yearly immunizations against this respiratory virus

23 - If you get chlamydia from your bird, you might have this

50 Step 1 Potpourri

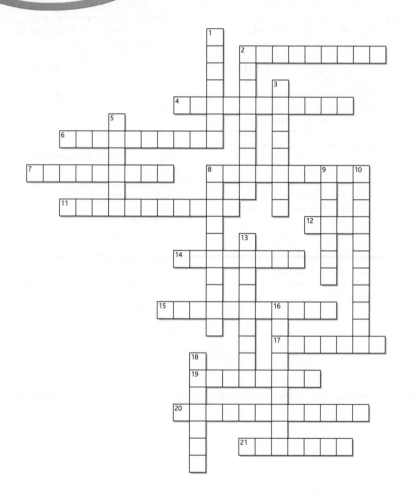

Across:

2 - Mediator released during mast cell activation that directly increases vascular permeability

4 - Term for movement of white blood cells to the periphery of the microcirculation

6 - If you ever see a pheochromocytoma, recall that it is a tumor of these cells in the adrenal medulla

7 - Proteinuria, edema, hypoalbuminemia, hyperlipidemia: _____ syndrome

8 - Made up of nine tubular triplets, these help with spindle formation

11 - Enzyme that protects red blood cells from in vivo generated hydrogen peroxide: _____ peroxidase

12 - Cholera infection causes massive diarrhea via a mechanism increasing levels of this in the intestines (acronym)

14 - Increases plasma glucose by stimulating glycogenolysis and gluconeogenesis

15 - Treatment for lead poisoning

17 - Pathologic finding in the hippocampus of patients with Alzheimer disease: Neurofibrillary _____

19 - Patients taking drug X have a risk of death of 10% while patients taking drug Y have a risk of death of 5%; 50% is the _____ risk reduction

20 - Patients with retinoblastoma are at increased risk of developing this cancer

21 - Tumor associated with myasthenia gravis

Down:

1 - Zollinger-Ellison syndrome is characterized by overproduction of this

2 - Defense mechanism in which people or events are seen as entirely good or entirely bad

3 - Anticoagulant reversed by vitamin K

5 - Study design in which subjects are initially free of disease and followed over time to assess whether an exposure is associated with development of disease

8 - In a research study, a third factor that is associated with both the exposure and the outcome is called a _____

9 - Muscle that raises the soft palate during swallowing: _____ veli palatini

10 - Antimuscarinic used to prevent motion sickness

13 - Virus that causes shingles when reactivated (genus)

16 - Bitemporal hemianopia may signify a tumor in this gland

18 - Down syndrome: _____ 21

1 My Heart Skips a Beat (when I do this puzzle)

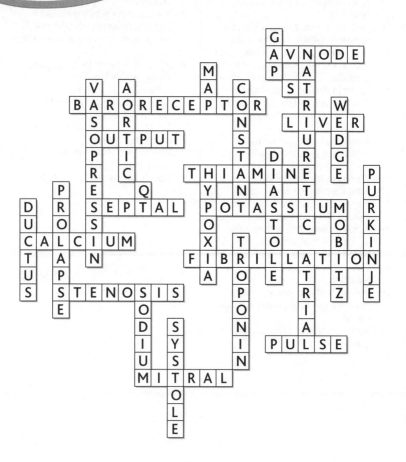

Across:

2 - Cardiac conduction velocity is slowest through this
AVNODE

8 - Classic ECG finding of acute MI: **ST** segment elevation

9 - Carotid massage works via a **BARO-RECEPTOR** to decrease heart rate

11 - This organ receives the largest share of cardiac output
LIVER

12 - Stroke volume × heart rate = cardiac **OUTPUT**

14 - Beriberi, which can cause dilated cardiomyopathy, is due to the deficiency of this
THIAMINE. *Dry beriberi affects nerves; wet beriberi affects the heart.*

20 - Fixed splitting of the second heart sound occurs in atrial **SEPTAL** defect

21 - Depolarization occurs when there is an influx of this into the myocardial cells
POTASSIUM. *Potassium is what determines the resting membrane potential of the cardiac cell.*

23 - Ventricular action potential plateau is due to an influx of **CALCIUM**

25 - Irregularly irregular rhythm with no discernible P waves = atrial **FIBRIL-LATION**. *This is a common arrhythmia you will see in older patients; increased risk of stroke.*

27 - Harsh crescendo–decrescendo systolic murmur could signify aortic **STENOSIS**

30 - Systolic pressure – diastolic pressure = **PULSE** pressure

31 - This valve closes during the first heart sound (S1)
MITRAL. *Tricuspid also closes during S1. Remember "MTAP."*

Down:

1 - Cardiac muscle cells are coupled each other by these junctions
GAP

3 - Atrial **NATRIURETIC** peptide is released when the atria "stretch" in response to increased volume

4 - 1/3 systolic pressure + 2/3 diastolic pressure (acronym)
MAP. *Mean arterial pressure.*

5 - Hormone that promotes water retention and direct arteriolar vasoconstriction
VASOPRESSIN

6 - The dicrotic notch of the cardiac cycle represents closure of the **AORTIC** valve

7 - Autoregulation keeps blood flow to an organ **CONSTANT**

10 - Pulmonary capillary **WEDGE** pressure measured with a catheter provides an estimate of left atrial pressure

13 - Cardiac relaxation phase
DIASTOLE

15 - **HYPOXIA** causes vasodilation in all organs except the lungs, where it causes vasoconstriction
This happens in the lungs so that the blood only goes to the areas that get oxygen.

16 - Cardiac conduction velocity is fastest through these fibers
PURKINJE

17 - The murmur of mitral valve **PROLAPSE** is described as a systolic crescendo murmur with a midsystolic click
MVP is the most common valve abnormality.

18 - Contraction of the left ventricle occurs during the **QT** interval
Right ventricle also contracts during this time.

19 - A patent **DUCTUS** arteriosus may be due to prematurity or congenital infection

22 - Progressive lengthening of PR interval until a beat (QRS) is dropped: **MOBITZ** type I second-degree block
Mobitz type I also known as Wenckebach. A Mobitz type II is when there are dropped beats (no QRS) without the progressive lengthening of the PR interval.

24 - This biomarker of MI lasts about 10 days
TROPONIN

26 - P-wave = **ATRIAL** depolarization

28 - The ventricular action potential begins when voltage-gated **SODIUM** channels open

29 - Cardiac contraction phase
SYSTOLE

2 A Bug's Life 1

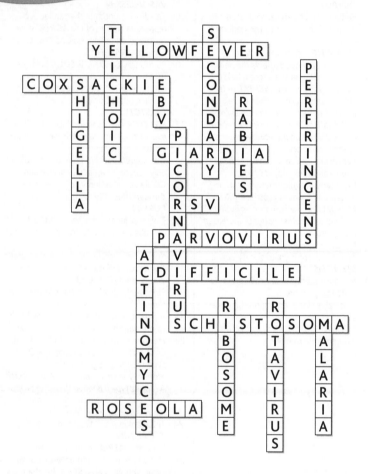

Across:

3 - If your febrile patient returning from South America has "black vomit" and jaundice, think this virus (two words) **YELLOW FEVER.** *A flavivirus transmitted by Aedes mosquito, mostly in South America and sub-Saharan Africa.*

5 - Hand-foot-and-mouth disease is caused by **COXSACKIE** virus type A *Coxsackie B: Guillain-Barre, pericarditis, myocarditis.*

10 - Protozoan genus that causes watery diarrhea **GIARDIA.** *Cryptosporidium is another, mostly affecting immunocompromised.*

11 - Major cause of viral pneumonia in infants (initials) **RSV.** *Respiratory syncytial virus.*

12 - **PARVOVIRUS** B19 causes erythema infectiosum (fifth disease) *Also causes aplastic crisis in sickle cell patients.*

14 - Antibiotic-associated diarrhea is usually caused by toxin from this organism (genus first letter and species) **CDIFFICILE.** *Toxin A (enterotoxin) and toxin B (cytotoxin) lead to pseudomembranous colitis.*

17 - Fluke associated with bladder cancer (genus) **SCHISTOSOMA.** *Schistosoma haematobium to be more precise.*

19 - Human herpesvirus (HHV)-6 causes this infantile illness **ROSEOLA.** *Also known as exanthem subitum; classically high fever for a few days followed by diffuse macular rash.*

Down:

1 - This cell membrane acid is unique to gram-positive organisms **TEICHOIC**

2 - A person with cough, fever, night sweat, and weight loss due to tuberculosis has this form **SECONDARY**

4 - Its toxin leads to gas gangrene: Clostridium **PERFRINGENS** (species) *Toxin is alpha-toxin, a phospholipase that causes myonecrosis.*

6 - One of the oxidase negative, lactose nonfermenting gram-negative rods (genus) **SHIGELLA.** *Salmonella and proteus are the two others.*

7 - Responsible for classic mononucleosis (initials) **EBV.** *Epstein Barr virus; positive heterophile antibody test.*

8 - Bats, raccoons, and skunks, oh my! This CNS infection has high fatality rate **RABIES.** *Long incubation period.*

9 - Hepatitis A belongs to this virus family **PICORNAVIRUS.** *Picornaviruses are small RNA viruses. Other ones are polio, echo, rhino, and coxsackie.*

13 - Gram-positive rods in branching filaments that resemble fungi and form sulfur granules (genus) **ACTINOMYCES.** *Normal oral flora but can lead to oral or facial infections.*

15 - Shigella inactivates the 60S one of these **RIBOSOME.** *And that is how it kills intestinal cells and causes diarrhea.*

16 - Major cause of infant diarrhea around the world and winter daycare diarrhea in US **ROTAVIRUS**

18 - If you see trophozoites and schizonts on a patient's blood smear, think **MALARIA**

3   A Rate-limiting Puzzle

Across:

5 - Stunted growth and cachexia in children due to prolonged deficiency of protein and calories
MARASMUS. *Remember that kwashiorkor is caused by protein deficiency with adequate calorie intake. Leads to stunted growth, anemia, and severe edema.*

6 - The rate-determining enzyme of glycolysis
PHOSPHOFRUCTOKINASE. *Technically PFK-1.*

8 - Byproducts of fatty acid metabolism, acetone can be detected in urine but this ketone body cannot: Beta-
HYDROXYBUTYRATE

13 - G6PD is the rate-limiting step in the **HMP** shunt (initials)

14 - Enzymes that stimulate release of arachidonic acid from phospholipids
PHOSPHOLIPASES

16 - **ISOCITRATE** dehydrogenase is the rate-limiting step of the tricarboxylic (citric) acid cycle

18 - Pyruvate is converted to this acid by dehydrogenase
LACTATE

19 - Primary source of energy for your brain (Hint: Not caffeine)
GLUCOSE

22 - Lipoxygenase acting on arachidonic acid results in these compounds
LEUKOTRIENES

24 - When DNA has had a rough day and it just needs to unwind, it relies on this (Hint: Not a glass of wine)
HELICASE. *Sometimes, I guess the biochemists run out of clever names.*

25 - HMG-CoA synthase is the rate-limiting step in **KETOGENESIS.** *Not to be confused with HMG-Co-A reductase – see #1 down.*

26 - One of four enzymes required for #12 down: Glucose-6-**PHOSPHATASE.**
Pyruvate carboxylase, phosphoenolpyruvate carboxykinase, and fructose 2,6-bisphosphatase are the others.

Down:

1 - **HMG-CoA** reductase regulates cholesterol synthesis (acronym)
Statin drugs work here.

2 - Rare disease due to the deficiency of glucocerebrosidase
GAUCHER. *Though rare, this is the most common lysosomal storage disease.*

3 - Rate-limiting step of fatty acid metabolism is the **CARNITINE** shuttle
Carnitine deficiency (which you will probably never see (1/100,000) except may be on an episode of House) leads to hypoketotic hypoglycemia.

4 - Substrate in the rate-limiting step in gluconeogenesis: Fructose-1,6-
BISPHOSPHATE

7 - Glycogen **PHOSPHORYLASE** is the rate-limiting step of glycogenolysis

9 - The receptor for insulin is part of a large family of **TYROSINE** kinase receptors

10 - A noncompetitive **INHIBITOR** has no effect on substrate binding and therefore no effect on Km
They can; however, decrease Vmax.

11 - Homocystinuria is caused by the deficiency of this synthase
CYSTATHIONE

12 - De novo synthesis of glucose
GLUCONEOGENESIS

15 - ALA synthase is the rate-limiting step in **HEME** synthesis

17 - Deficiency of hexosaminidase A leads to this disease
TAY-SACHS. *Cherry red spot on macula not to be confused with Niemann–Pick disease.*

20 - Carbamoyl phosphate synthetase I is the rate-limiting step of this cycle
UREA

21 - This enzyme seals the DNA deal
Nope, not "sealase" but good try.
LIGASE.

23 - Cleaves peptide bonds on the carboxyl side of lysine or arginine
TRYPSIN. *Trypsin is a pancreatic enzyme.*

4 How Many Psychiatrists Does it Take...?*

Yemeng Lu

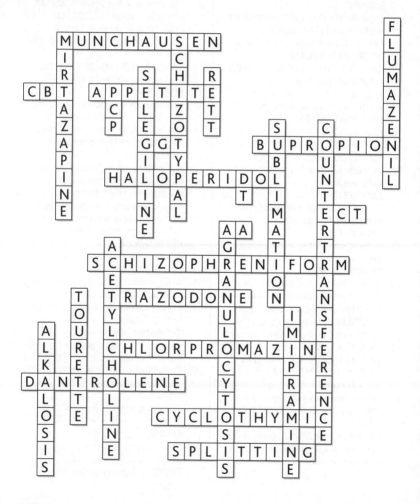

Across:

2 - Chronic factitious disorder: **_MUNCHAUSEN_** syndrome
Munchausen's by proxy is usually caretakers intentionally making their children sick. (Also, the name of Zooey Deschanel's band in the movie Yes Man.)

6 - Treatment of panic disorder that addresses dysfunctional emotions and maladaptive behaviors (acronym)
CBT. *It focuses on examining the relationships between thoughts, feelings, and behaviors. We could all benefit from some...*

7 - "A" in SIG E CAPS stands for **_APPETITE_**

11 - A sensitive indicator of alcohol use (laboratory marker, acronym)
GGT. *Another indicator is elevated MCV.*

12 - Antidepressant that girls on the eating disorder unit should avoid
BUPROPION. *Their seizure threshold is already pretty low.*

13 - High-potency neuroleptic known for causing EPS
HALOPERIDOL

15 - Treatment of choice for refractory major depressive disorder with the major adverse side effect being amnesia (acronym)
ECT. *Controlled seizures in anesthetized patients.*

16 - The tried-and-true best relapse prevention for alcohol dependence (acronym)
_AA_. *"Hi, My name is Fred... ""HI FRED"*

18 - Symptoms similar to schizophrenia, but for only 3 months
SCHIZOPHRENIFORM. *<1 month of symptoms is brief psychotic disorder.*

20 - Antidepressant known to cause priapism
TRAZODONE

23 - Low-potency antipsychotic associated with corneal deposits
CHLORPROMAZINE. *While thioridazine is associated with retinal deposits.*

24 - Your patient on a neuroleptic develops a fever, muscle rigidity, has unstable vitals and myoglobinuria. You treat with
DANTROLENE
Neuroleptic malignant syndrome is a life-threatening neurologic emergency with 10% to 20% mortality. Bromocriptine can be used as well.

25 - Milder form of bipolar disorder characterized by dysthymia and hypomania:
CYCLOTHYMIC disorder
Has to be happening for at least 2 years for diagnosis.

26 - Defense mechanism that borderline patients use: Believing that people are either all good or all bad
SPLITTING

Down:

1 - Treatment for benzodiazepine overdose **_FLUMAZENIL_**. *Competitive GABA receptor antagonist.*

2 - Antidepressant of choice for little old ladies who need to sleep better and gain weight **_MIRTAZAPINE_**. *An alpha-2 antagonist that causes sedation and increased appetite.*

3 - Think hard! You probably have a friend who has very odd beliefs about magic powers, has eccentric behaviors, and is socially awkward; he most likely has **_SCHIZO-TYPAL_** personality disorder
Not to be confused with schizophreniform (see #18 across), schizoid, or schizophrenia.

4 - MAO-B inhibitor used in Parkinson disease **_SELEGILINE_**. *An MAO-B specific inhibitor.*

5 - Stereotyped hand-wringing in a previously healthy 4-year-old girl who can no longer speak: **_RETT_** syndrome

8 - Intoxication with **_PCP_** produces impulsiveness, belligerence, nystagmus, psychosis (acronym)
Stands for phencyclidine and known as "angel dust" on the streets.

9 - A CEO of a large bank who is frustrated at work and releases his energy in the gym demonstrates a defense mechanism called **_SUBLIMATION_**

10 - The psychiatrist who gets upset at the patient for substance abuse because his own mother recently passed away from alcoholic liver cirrhosis is exhibiting **_COUNTERTRANSFERENCE_**

14 - A severe alcohol withdrawal (acronym) **_DT_**

16 - Your patient on clozapine requires weekly WBC monitoring to check for **_AGRANU-LOCYTOSIS_**

17 - The neurotransmitter thought to be decreased in Alzheimer dementia **_ACETYLCHOLINE_**. *Therefore, you use Donepezil, galantamine, or rivastigmine (acetylcholinesterase inhibitors) for treatment.*

19 - One out of five patients with this syndrome has coprolalia
TOURETTE. *Coprolalia (aka potty mouth) does not happen in all with Tourette.*

21 - Jimmy is 12 and still wets the bed and has failed the bed alarm; let us try this medication
IMIPRAMINE. *Also can be used as an adjunct for cancer pain and PTSD.*

22 - pH disturbance in bulimia nervosa patients: Metabolic **_ALKALOSIS_**
Chronic emesis (losing HCl).

5 What's the Antidote?

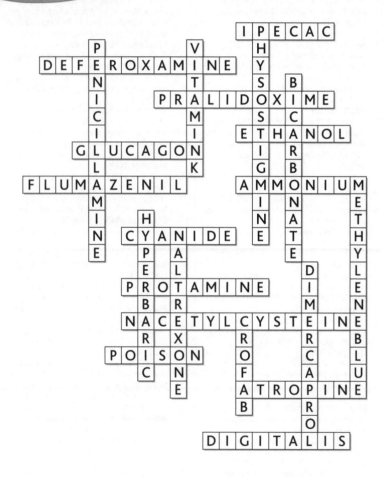

Across:

1 - Induces vomiting: Syrup of **IPECAC**
This is no longer recommended.

5 - Iron toxicity
DEFEROXAMINE

7 - Used with #21 across
PRALIDOXIME

8 - Methanol ingestion
ETHANOL. *That is right – treat methanol (and ethylene glycol [antifreeze]) with regular old alcohol (and possibly dialysis). Fomepizole is now preferred 1st-line therapy, with ethanol used if fomepizole is not available.*

9 - Beta-blocker toxicity
GLUCAGON

10 - Benzodiazepine overdose
FLUMAZENIL

11 - Amphetamine toxicity: **AMMONIUM** chloride

14 - Kit for this poisoning includes amyl nitrite and thiosulfate
CYANIDE

17 - Reverses heparin
PROTAMINE

18 - Acetaminophen overdose
N-ACETYLCYSTEINE

20 - 1-800-222-1222: **POISON** control number in US

21 - Insecticide (organophosphate) poisoning
ATROPINE

22 - Anti-dig Fab fragments are used for toxicity from this
DIGITALIS. *Also pay attention to potassium level.*

Down:

2 - Anticholinergic toxicity
PHYSOSTIGMINE

3 - Copper toxicity
PENICILLAMINE

4 - Reverses warfarin
VITAMINK

6 - Aspirin overdose: Sodium **BICARBONATE**
To alkalinize the urine.

12 - Methemoglobin (two words)
METHYLENE BLUE

13 - CO poisoning: **HYPERBARIC** oxygen

15 - Opiate overdose
NALTREXONE

16 - Mercury toxicity
DIMERCAPROL. *"Mad hatter disease" is so-named because the mercury used in making felt hats was toxic, leading to the symptoms Johnny Depp portrayed in Alice in Wonderland.*

19 - Rattlesnake bite (trade name)
CROFAB. *Made famous by Dr. Sean Bush on "Venom ER."*

6 Your Microtubules are Showing

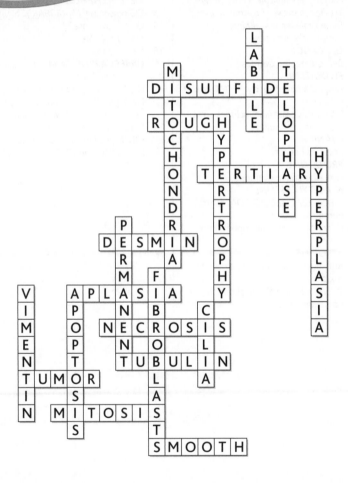

Across:

4 - Kinds of bonds important to maintain #8 across
DISULFIDE

5 - Form of endoplasmic reticulum; that is, the site of synthesis of secretory proteins
ROUGH. *Also site of synthesis of certain enzymes.*

8 - Final structure of most proteins is the **TERTIARY** structure

10 - Muscle cell stain
DESMIN

13 - Term for complete failure of cell production
APLASIA

15 - Irreversible cell injury/death
NECROSIS

16 - Microtubules are made up of dimers of alpha- and beta-**TUBULIN**
Microtubules are the site of action of several drugs including mebendazole, vincristine, colchicines, and others.

17 - Rb and p53 are **TUMOR** suppressors
They inhibit G_1 to S-phase progression; mutations in tumor suppressor lead to unchecked cell growth; that is, a tumor.

18 - Consists of prophase, metaphase, and anaphase
MITOSIS

19 - Form of endoplasmic reticulum that is site of steroid synthesis
SMOOTH. *"S" in smooth, "s" in steroids; also site of detoxification.*

Down:

1 - Rapidly dividing cells that never go to G_0
LABILE. *Examples are skin cells, hair follicles, intestinal lining, and bone marrow.*

2 - When these are damaged, cytochrome c and H^+ are released
MITOCHONDRIA

3 - Phase missing from clue #18 across
TELOPHASE

6 - Increase in the size of an organ due to an increase in the size of the cells
HYPERTROPHY. *For example left ventricular hypertrophy.*

7 - Increase in the size of an organ due to an increase in the number of cells
HYPERPLASIA. *For example, benign prostatic hyperplasia.*

9 - Cells that stay in G_0 and regenerate from stem cells
PERMANENT. *Examples are neurons, red blood cells, skeletal muscle cells, and cardiac muscle cells.*

11 - Collagen-making cells
FIBROBLASTS. *Collagen is the most abundant protein in the body.*

12 - Connective tissue stain
VIMENTIN

13 - Programmed cell death
APOPTOSIS

14 - These have a 9 + 2 arrangement of microtubules
CILIA. *Kartagener syndrome is immotile cilia due to a defect in the dynein arm.*

7   Where is My Mind?

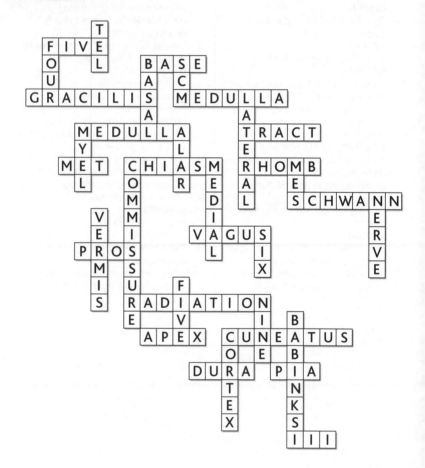

Across:

2 - Herniation of the L4–L5 disc would produce a lumbar radiculopathy
FIVE. Clinically manifest as a foot drop, weakness to dorsiflexion, pain on dorsum of foot.

3 - High-frequency cochlea
BASE

5 - Fascicle of the lower limb
GRACILIS. Forms the medial portion of the posterior columns.

6 - Site of decussation: Posterior columns
MEDULLA

8 - Site of decussation: Corticospinal tract
MEDULLA. (Yep, it is here twice!)

10 - Unilateral hemianopsia lesion: Optic
TRACT

11 - *MET*encephalon (forms pons/cerebellum)
Part of the rhombencephalon.

12 - Bitemporal hemianopsia lesion: Optic
CHIASM
The nasal fibers cross in the chiasm, the temporal fibers do not, thus the temporal fibers (which see the nasal part of the field) are unaffected.

14 - *RHOMB*encephalon (hindbrain)
Forms the medulla, pons, cerebellum.

16 - Myelinator cell
SCHWANN. Schwann cells produce myelin which ensheaths axons and speeds conduction.

19 - Cranial nerve assessed by gag reflex
VAGUS

21 - *PROS*encephalon (forebrain)
Forms the diencephalon and the telencephalon.

23 - Unilateral quadrantanopsia lesion: Optic
RADIATION

26 - Low-frequency cochlea
APEX

27 - Fascicle of the upper limb
CUNEATUS. Forms the lateral portion of the posterior columns.

28 - *DURA* mater: Outermost layer of meninges
Latin for "hard mother."

29 - *PIA* mater: Innermost layer of meninges
Latin for "soft mother."

30 - Cranial nerve for pupils
III. Also controls all of the extraocular muscles except for superior oblique and lateral rectus.

Down:

1 - *TEL*encephalon (forms cerebral hemispheres)
Part of the prosencephalon.

2 - Superior oblique cranial nerve
FOUR. Moves the eye downward and internally rotates.

3 - Plate of neural tube that forms motor nerves
BASAL

4 - Muscle innervated by CN XI
SCM. Sternocleidomastoid, responsible for rotating the head in the contralateral direction.

7 - Geniculate body for light
LATERAL. Remember the Lets go together (light and lateral).

8 - *MYEL*encephalon (forms medulla)
Part of the rhombencephalon.

9 - Plate of the neural tube that forms sensory nerves
ALAR

12 - Site of decussation: Spinothalamic tract
COMMISSURE

13 - Geniculate body for music
MEDIAL. Remember the M's go together (music and medial).

15 - *MES*encephalon (midbrain)
Contains tectum, tegmentum, cerebral peduncles, responsible for sight/sound, motor control, and level of alertness.

17 - Unilateral blindness lesion: Optic
NERVE
Complete loss of entire visual field on the affected side.

18 - Herniation of this part of the cerebellum seen in Arnold–Chiari malformation
VERMIS

20 - Longest cranial nerve in the brain
SIX. And most susceptible to injury as a result, with CN VI palsy being the most common CN palsy.

22 - Herniation of the C4–C5 disc would produce a cervical radiculopathy
FIVE. Clinically manifest as deltoid weakness, and numbness over the shoulder.

24 - Taste to the posterior third of the tongue by this cranial nerve
NINE. CN IX also innervates the stylopharyngeus muscle.

25 - Upper motor neuron "sign"
BABINSKI. Defined as extension of the big toe.

27 - Macular sparing lesion: Optic *CORTEX*
On the posterior cerebellum. Injury may be due to a posterior cerebral artery stroke.

8 Ain't Life Gland?

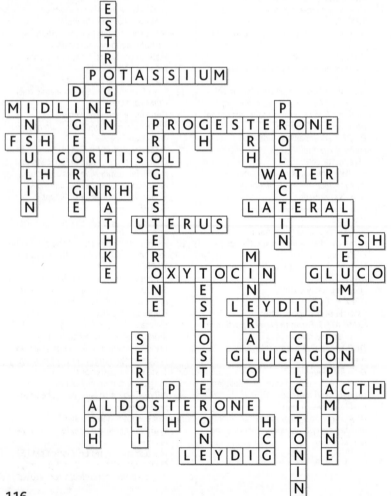

Across:

2 - #31 across also increases renal secretion of this electrolyte
POTASSIUM. *This is why aldosterone-antagonists such as spironolactone are "potassium-sparing."*

4 - Thyroglossal duct cysts are found midline/lateral
MIDLINE. *Just like the thyroid is in the midline.*

7 - Responsible for breast development during puberty
PROGESTERONE

10 - Promotes growth of ovarian follicle (acronym)
FOLLICLE STIMULATING HORMONE (FSH). *Released from the anterior pituitary.*

11 - Systemic anti-inflammatory effects, immuno-suppression, elevation of blood glucose
CORTISOL

12 - Triggers ovulation
LUTEINIZING HORMONE (LH). *The "LH surge" occurs at midcycle.*

13 - #31 down increases reabsorption of this molecule in the distal tubule
WATER

14 - Triggers LH/FSH release (acronym)
GNRH (GONADOTROPIN RELEASING HORMONE). *Released from the hypothalamus.*

16 - Branchial cleft cysts are found midline/lateral
LATERAL

18 - #21 across stimulates contractions of this smooth muscle organ
UTERUS. *Responsible for labor.*

19 - Stimulates release of thyroid hormone (acronym)
TSH (THYROID STIMULATING HORMONE). *Released from anterior pituitary.*

21 - Stimulates milk letdown
OXYTOCIN. *Released from posterior pituitary.*

23 - **GLUCO**-corticoids are released from adrenal cortical zona fasciculate
Cortisol is the primary glucocorticoid.

24 - Testosterone is produced in these cells in the testes
LEYDIG

28 - Pancreatic hormone which increases blood glucose
GLUCAGON. *Promotes glycogenolysis and gluconeogenesis.*

30 - Promotes secretion of adrenal cortical hormones
ACTH (ADRENOCORTICOTROPIC HORMONE). *Released from the anterior pituitary.*

31 - Increases renal retention of Na⁺
ALDOSTERONE

33 - LH acts on these cells in testes and increases testosterone production
LEYDIG. *Remember LH acts on Leydig cells.*

Down:

1 - Causes proliferation of endometrium
ESTROGEN

3 - Congenital absence of the parathyroids may be seen in this syndrome
DIGEORGE. *The CATCH-22 syndrome: Cardiac abnormalities, abnormal facies, thymic aplasia, cleft palate, hypocalcemia, and hypoparathyroidism, on chromosome 22.*

5 - Pancreatic hormone which decreases blood glucose
INSULIN. *Synthesized by the pancreatic beta cells.*

6 - Stimulates milk production
PROLACTIN. *Galactorrhea may be a sign of a prolactinoma.*

7 - Promotes transition from proliferative to secretory endometrium
PROGESTERONE. *Produced by the corpus luteum.*

8 - Promotes increase in lean body mass (acronym)
GH (GROWTH HORMONE). *The liver produces insulin-like growth factor 1 in response to GH.*

9 - Promotes release of TSH from the thyroid and prolactin from the anterior pituitary (acronym)
TRH (THYROID RELEASING HORMONE). *Released from the hypothalamus.*

15 - Craniopharyngioma forms from the remnants of this embryologic pouch
RATHKE

17 - LH promotes formation of the corpus **LUTEUM**
Hence the "luteal phase" of the menstrual cycle.

20 - **MINERALO**-corticoids are released from adrenal cortical zona glomerulosa
Aldosterone is a major mineralocorticoid.

22 - Triggers spermatogenesis
TESTOSTERONE

25 - FSH acts on these cells to promote sperm maturation
SERTOLI

26 - "Tones down" calcium in the blood
CALCITONIN. *Produced by C-cells in the thyroid.*

27 - Inhibits prolactin release
DOPAMINE

29 - Increases serum calcium, "trashes phosphate" (acronym)
PTH (PARATHYROID HORMONE). *Also known as "phosphate trashing hormone."*

31 - Causes constriction of vascular smooth muscle through its V1 receptor (acronym)
ADH (ANTIDIURETIC HORMONE). *Also known as vasopressin. Released from the posterior pituitary.*

32 - Maintains the corpus luteum if implantation occurs (acronym)
HCG (HUMAN CHORIONIC GONADOTROPIN). *Produced by the placenta.*

9 Clinical Scramble

LORIPAUY

P	O	L	Y	U	R	I	**A**

RUGBYDIEL

G	L	Y	**B**	U	R	I	D	**E**

GAPYOLIPHA

P	O	L	Y	P	H	A	G	**I**	A

TENMORFIM

M	**E**	**T**	F	O	R	M	I	N

OPLIDAYSIP

P	O	L	Y	**D**	I	P	**S**	I	A

ANSWER: _____ **DIABETES** _____

Notes

10 Let's Get PUMPED!

Yemeng Lu

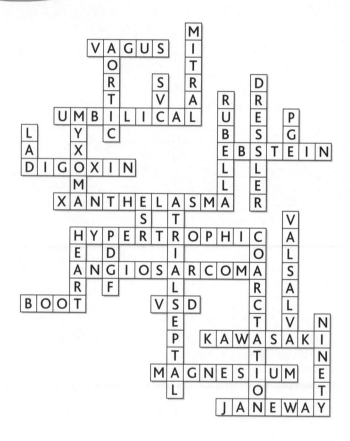

Across:

2 - Enlargement of the left atrium can produce hoarseness due to the compression of a nerve; that is, a branch of the **VAGUS** nerve
Recurrent laryngeal nerve is a branch of vagus.

7 - Fetal vessel with the highest oxygenation: **UMBILICAL** vein
It brings oxygenated blood from the placenta to the fetus.

11 - A pregnant 25-year-old woman with well-controlled bipolar type I mood disorder is at risk for having a child with **EBSTEIN** anomaly of the heart
It is caused by lithium use, characterized by a hypoplastic right ventricle, and tricuspid leaflets displaced into the right ventricle.

12 - Medication that works by inhibiting Na/K ATPase and increases cardiac contractility **DIGOXIN**

13 - **XANTHELASMA** can be associated with familial hypercholesterolemia and cholesterol deposited underneath the skin of the eyelid

17 - The murmur of **HYPERTROPHIC** cardiomyopathy increases with the Valsalva maneuver

20 - Your patient who works at a plastic manufacturing company producing vinyl products is at risk for developing **ANGIOSARCOMA**

21 - Tetralogy of falot will likely result in a **BOOT**-shaped cardiac silhouette

22 - The most common congenital cardiac anomaly (acronym)
VSD. Ventricular septal defect.

24 - IVIG (which evidently can cost $10,000) + aspirin is the treatment of choice for kids with **KAWASAKI** disease
It is characterized by conjunctivitis, lymphadenitis, fever, skin desquamation, strawberry tongue.

25 - Treatment of choice for a patient with ventricular tachy with shifting sinusoidal waveforms on ECG
MAGNESIUM. *Torsades de pointes is characterized by shifting sinusoidal waveforms, and treated with Mg.*

26 - These lesions are nontender, erythematous, macular/nodular on the palm and soles and pathognomonic for infective endocarditis
JANEWAY. *Splinter hemorrhages, Roth spots, and Osler nodes are also associated with bacterial endocarditis.*

Down:

1 - The QRS complex in ECG corresponds to the closing of the **MITRAL** valve

3 - Your patient unintentionally bobs his head with every heartbeat; he likely has pathology in his **AORTIC** valve (P.S. There is no "Call Me Maybe" playing in the room)
De Musset sign is rhythmic nodding of the head in synchrony with HR, which results from aortic regurgitation.

4 - Embryonic structure: Right common cardinal vein and right anterior cardinal vein give rise to the **SVC** (acronym)
Superior vena cava.

5 - Your 65-year-old patient, 4 weeks post an acute-MI presents with sudden, sharp, pleuritic, and positional chest pain likely has **DRESSLER** syndrome
It is an autoimmune fibrinous pericarditis that occurs 4 to 6 weeks post MI.

6 - A continuous machine-like murmur heard in an infant can result from congenital **RUBELLA** infection
It can lead to patent ductus arteriorosis.

8 - "Ball-valve" obstruction in the left atrium
MYXOMA. *It is the most common adult primary cardiac tumor.*

9 - For babies with transposition of the great artery, this agent can be used to keep a fetal vessel open in order to improve oxygenation (acronym)
PGE. *Transposition of the great vessels is not compatible with life unless a shunt is present to allow adequate mixing of blood (such as a VSD, PDA, or patent forament ovale).*

10 - Artery that supplies the apex and anterior septum of the heart (acronym)
LAD

14 - This inflammatory marker is often elevated in patients with temporal arteritis (acronym)
ESR

15 - You hear a split S2 sound that does not vary with respiration in a child and suspect **ATRIAL SEPTAL** defect (two words)
Fixed splitting is seen in ASD due to left to right shunting.

16 - You tell a patient, "Bear down like you are having a bowel movement (but DON'T!)" to perform the **VALSALVA** maneuver

17 - This organ is super efficient in extracting O_2 – 100% and has largest arteriovenous O_2 difference
HEART

18 - The pathogenesis of atherosclerosis involves migration of the smooth muscle cell which is influenced by the mitogen/chemoattractant **PDGF** (acronym)
Platelet-derived growth factor (PDGF) is a mitogen and chemoattractant for vascular smooth muscle cells.

19 - Your 48-year-old patient who has BP of 160/90 on the right arm and 170/92 on the left arm and has no peripheral pedal pulses likely has **COARCTATION** of the aorta
Asymmetric upper extremity blood pressure is a common finding in aortic coarctation.

23 - Approximate pulse pressure of a patient with a diastolic BP of 60 and MAP of 90
NINETY. *MAP = 2/3 diastolic BP + 1/3 systolic BP, Pulse pressure = systolic – diastolic.*

11 A Short Round of Chemo (Drugs)

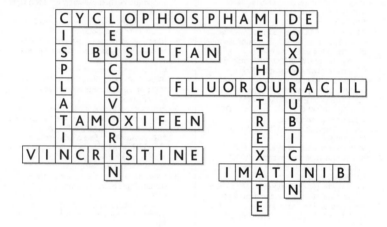

Across:

1 - Alkylating agent used to prevent transplant rejection as well as for some cancers
CYCLOPHOSPHAMIDE

5 - Alkylating agent used for leukemia; classic toxicity is pulmonary fibrosis
BUSULFAN

6 - 5-<u>**FLUOROURACIL**</u> is a pyrimidine analog that binds folate, used topically to treat basal cell carcinoma

7 - Competitively binds estrogen receptors, used to treat estrogen-receptor + breast cancers
TAMOXIFEN

8 - Depolymerizes microtubules so spindle cannot form
VINCRISTINE

9 - Trade name Gleevec, this tyrosine kinase inhibitor is used to treat CML
IMATINIB

Down:

1 - Another alkylating agent, used for bladder cancer, can damage the acoustic nerves
CISPLATIN

2 - Given as a rescue medication to reverse bone marrow suppression
LEUCOVORIN

3 - Dihydrofolate reductase inhibitor used to treat leukemia/lymphoma, rheumatoid arthritis, psoriasis, and even ectopic pregnancy
METHOTREXATE

4 - Used for Hodgkin's lymphoma and myeloma, this agent's classic adverse effect is cardiotoxicity (leading to heart failure)
DOXORUBICIN

12 GI Know that Part

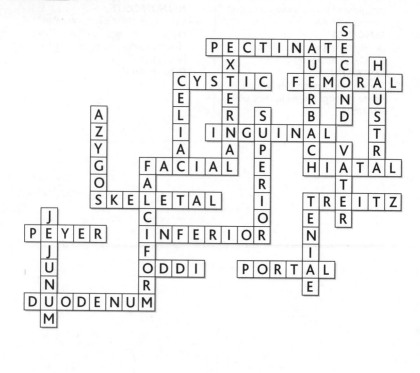

Across:

2 - Divides upper and lower anal canal: ***PECTINATE*** line
External hemorrhoids are from below the line (and internal [painless] are from above).

6 - The ***CYSTIC*** duct combines with the common hepatic duct to form the common bile duct

7 - Hernia below the inguinal ligament lateral to pubic tubercle ***FEMORAL***

10 - Hesselbach's triangle is formed by the inferior epigastric artery, the ***INGUINAL*** ligament, and the lateral border of the rectus abdominal
Direct inguinal hernias protrude through this triangle.

12 - This cranial nerve courses through the parotid ***FACIAL***. *CN 7.*

13 - If your stomach is riding up through your diaphragm, you have a ***HIATAL*** hernia

14 - Proximal one-third of esophagus is composed of this type of muscle ***SKELETAL***. *The distal one-third is smooth, and the middle is mixed.*

15 - The ligament of ***TREITZ*** connects fourth part of the duodenum to the diaphragm near the splenic flexure
We talk about GI bleeds being proximal or distal to the ligament of Treitz, which separates upper from lower GI bleeding.

17 - Lymphoid tissue in the lamina propia of small intestine: ***PEYER*** patches

18 - Direct hernia passes medial to the ***INFERIOR*** epigastric artery
See also #10 across.

19 - Regulates release of bile into the duodenum: Sphincter of ***ODDI***

20 - The superior mesenteric vein and splenic vein join to form the ***PORTAL*** vein

21 - The gastroduodenal artery is just posterior to the first part of this ***DUODENUM***. *So beware a perforated duodenal ulcer.*

Down:

1 - #11 down opens into the ***SECOND*** part of the duodenum

3 - The ***EXTERNAL*** anal sphincter is composed of striated muscle

4 - Enteric plexus between the longitudinal and circular layers of GI tract ***AUERBACH***

5 - "Walls" in the colon ***HAUSTRA***. *Easily seen by colonoscopy.*

6 - This artery, via branches off its trunk, supplies blood to stomach, liver, gallbladder, pancreas, and spleen ***CELIAC***

8 - This vein runs up the right side of the thoracic vertebral column providing an alternate path for blood to get into the right atrium (e.g., if IVC is blocked)
AZYGOS. *"Azygos" means unpaired.*

9 - This branch of the abdominal aorta comes off at L1: ***SUPERIOR*** mesenteric artery

11 - The pancreatic duct and common bile duct empty into the duodenum through the ampulla of ***VATER***
Note not spelled the same as the famous Darth's name.

12 - Ligament that connects liver to anterior abdominal wall
FALCIFORM. *This is a remnant of the fetal umbilical vein.*

15 - The three longitudinal bands of smooth muscle in the large intestine: ***TENIAE*** coli

16 - Where you will find your plicae circularis (if you look hard enough) ***JEJUNUM***

13 Private Parts

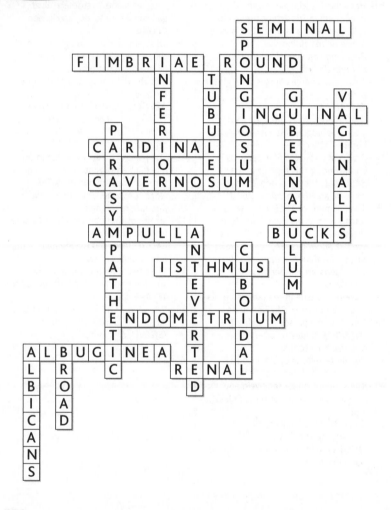

Across:

1 - Sperm are stored in these prior to ejaculation: **_SEMINAL_** vesicles
This is why a vasectomy takes about 3 months before it is effective: These have to clear.

2 - Finger-like projections at the opening of the fallopian tubes
FIMBRIAE

4 - These run from the uterine fundus to the labia majora: **_ROUND_** ligaments
A common site of pain in pregnancy as the uterus enlarges.

8 - Distal 1/3 of genital lymphatic drainage is via the superficial **_INGUINAL_** nodes
Enlarged inguinal nodes sometimes accompany sexually transmitted infections.

10 - Uterine vessels are contained in this ligament
CARDINAL

11 - Pair of sponge-like regions of erectile tissue within the penis dorsally: Corpus **_CAVERNOSUM_**

12 - Portion of uterine tube that is usual site of fertilization
AMPULLA

14 - Membranous layer of superficial fascia of penis: **_BUCK'S_** fascia

16 - Longest segment of uterine (fallopian) tubes
ISTHMUS

17 - Inner lining of the uterus
ENDOMETRIUM

18 - Layer of connective tissue covering the testicles: Tunica **_ALBUGINEA_**

20 - The left testicle's venous drainage is from the left gonadal vein to the left **_RENAL_** vein
See Private Parts Path puzzle for why this is relevant.

Down:

1 - Urethra runs through the corpus **_SPONGIOSUM_** of the penis which also forms the glans

3 - Ureter is posterior and **_INFERIOR_** to uterine artery
"Water runs under the bridge."

5 - Spermatogenesis occurs in the seminiferous
TUBULES

6 - Everyone's favorite embryonic structure, this aids in the descent of the gonads
GUBERNACULUM. *Admit it – when you first heard this word you called your friend a gubernaculum.*

7 - The serous covering of the testes: tunica **_VAGINALIS_**

9 - Erection is enabled by the **_PARASYM-PATHETIC_** nervous system
"Point (para-) before you shoot (sympa-)."

13 - Normal position of uterus
ANTEVERTED

15 - Ovary epithelium is simple **_CUBOIDAL_**

18 - Regressed form of the corpus luteum: Corpus **_ALBICANS_**

19 - This "ligament" connects the uterus, uterine tubes, and ovaries to the pelvic side wall
BROAD

14 This Puzzle Makes My Brain Hurt

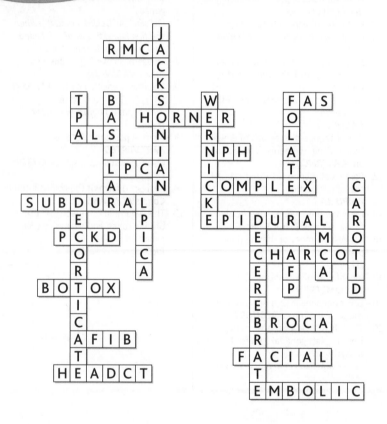

Across:

2 - Artery (acronym): L hemiparesis, L facial droop, L sided neglect
RMCA. Right middle cerebral artery. *Neglect should always prompt you to consider R-sided lesions—in this case, the R parietal lobe supplied by the middle cerebral artery.*

6 - Most common cause of mental retardation (acronym)
FAS. Fetal alcohol syndrome. *Characteristic facial abnormalities include small palpebral fissures, smooth philtrum, and thin vermilion border.*

7 - Syndrome of ptosis, anhydrosis, flushing, miosis
HORNER ('s) SYNDROME. *Seen in injuries to the ipsilateral sympathetic chain, often the result of trauma, or tumor (classically the Pancoast tumor).*

8 - Debilitating disease of upper and lower motor neurons (acronym)
ALS. Amyotrophic lateral sclerosis *or Lou Gehrig disease. Also famously affects physicist Stephen Hawking.*

9 - "Wacky, wobbly, and wet" disease (acronym)
NPH. Normal pressure hydrocephalus. *Classic triad of dementia, gait ataxia, and urinary incontinence.*

10 - Artery (acronym): R homonymous hemianopsia
LPCA. Left posterior cerebral artery. *Supplies the visual cortex.*

11 - Indicates that a seizure lead to loss of consciousness
COMPLEX

13 - Hematoma with a concave shape
SUBDURAL. *Caused by disruption of bridging veins. Think of this in an elder with a fall.*

16 - Hematoma with a lucid interval
EPIDURAL. *Caused by disruption of the middle meningeal artery, rapidly fatal if untreated.*

19 - A subarachnoid hemorrhage may be seen in patients with this disease (acronym)
PCKD (Yes, it's a tricky abbreviation) Polycystic kidney disease. *Associated with berry aneurysms in the brain.*

20 - Multiple sclerosis triad of nystagmus, scanning speech, intention tremor
CHARCOT (triad)

22 - Toxin that wrinkles ACh release
BOTOX. *Classically found in honey. Also used cosmetically to alleviate stigmata of aging.*

23 - Form of expressive aphasia
BROCA. *Comprehension is spared.*

24 - Cardiac arrhythmia responsible for majority of cardioembolic stroke (short form)
AFIB. Atrial fibrillation. *Absence of strong atrial contraction leads to venous stasis and atrial clot formation.*

25 - Cranial nerve affected in Bell's palsy
FACIAL (CN VII). *Clinically presents as facial drop without forehead sparing.*

26 - Imaging study obtained STAT with any suspected stroke
HEAD CT. *Rules out intracranial hemorrhage, helps differentiate ischemic versus hemorrhagic stroke.*

27 - Most common mechanism of stroke
EMBOLIC. *Which leads to the most common type of stroke: Ischemic.*

Down:

1 - Marching seizure (or perhaps moonwalking?)
JACKSONIAN. *So called because the seizure activity moves (marches) from one body area to another. Michael Jackson invented the moonwalk.*

3 - "Clot busting" drug indicated for some strokes (acronym)
TPA. Tissue plasminogen activator.

4 - Artery: Drop attack and vertigo
BASILAR. *Vertigo is due to loss of blood supply to the CN VIII nucleus.*

5 - Form of fluent aphasia, sometimes a "word salad"
WERNICKE('s). *Comprehension and repetition affected as well.*

6 - Women need adequate quantities of this vitamin to prevent neural tube defects
FOLATE

12 - Artery: Amaurosis fugax
CAROTID. *Greek for "fleeting darkness," a term to describe a transient monocular vision loss, caused by loss of flow through the ophthalmic artery, a distal branch of the internal carotid.*

14 - Posturing characterized by flexion
DECORTICATE. *Seen in injury to the hemispheres, internal capsule, and thalamus.*

15 - Artery (acronym): L facial sensory loss, R body sensory loss
LPICA. Left posterior inferior cerebellar artery. *Known as the lateral medullary syndrome or Wallenberg syndrome.*

17 - Posturing characterized by extension
DECEREBRATE. *Seen in brainstem injury.*

18 - Artery (acronym): R hemiparesis, R facial droop, aphasia
LMCA. Left middle cerebral artery. *99% of patients are L hemisphere dominant, and language is affected.*

21 - Serum marker elevated in neural tube defects (acronym)
AFP. Alpha fetoprotein. *Part of the "quad" or "tetra" screen for trisomy 18, 21, and neural tube defects.*

15 FOOSH!*

```
                              F
        T R E N D E L E N B U R G
          R     L             U
          A     E             Y
          D     X             O
          I     O       C O L L E S
          A     R       A       S
          L   T   B O X E R S
              H   X   A R P
        U P P E R   C A L C A N E U S
          E   A   R   A L     L
          R   D   C       N
        S C O L I O S I S     N
        N   N   A     C   T I B I A L
      G L U T E A L       E       R
        F   A L       T   R
        F   L     C   E   E     L
      H B         A V A S C U L A R
    P A L L O R   P   M       T
    M     X   M   I   M I D D L E
    A C L     E   T   N       R
    T         D S C A P H O I D   A
  M E R A L G I A     T   R       L
            A         E
            N
```

*Fall on outstretched hand – a common mechanism of injury

Across:

2 - When standing on one leg, the opposite hip drops: **_TRENDELEN-BURG_** sign

6 - Distal radius fracture with dorsal displacement of hand **_COLLES_**

7 - Fracture of the fifth metacarpal is also known as a **_BOXER'S_** fracture

8 - Injury to **_UPPER_** trunk of brachial plexus can lead to waiter's tip
Also called Erb–Duchenne.

11 - Jumping off your roof might cause you to fracture one
CALCANEUS. *Calcaneal fracture can be associated with lumbar fracture as well.*

13 - Lateral curvature of spine **_SCOLIOSIS_**

14 - Ability to plantar flex our foot is courtesy of the **_TIBIAL_** nerve

15 - A positive #2 across can indicate injury to superior **_GLUTEAL_** nerve

19 - An overlooked scaphoid fracture can result in **_AVASCULAR_** necrosis
Splint if unsure.

20 - One of the 6 P's of compartment syndrome
PALLOR. *Pain, parasthesias, paralysis, pulselessness, and poikilothermia (cold) are the others.*

22 - If you just fell down while doing this puzzle and fractured your clavicle, the most likely site is the **_MIDDLE_** one-third

23 - Positive anterior drawer test = torn **_ACL_** (acronym)
Anterior cruciate ligament.

24 - Tenderness in #13 down after a fall on an outstretched hand suggests **_SCAPHOID_** fracture
Even if you do not see it on x-ray, splint it for 2 weeks.

25 - **_MERALGIA_** paresthetica can result from injury to lateral femoral cutaneous nerve
Can be simply due to compression from a thick wallet (a problem I wish I had!) or tight clothes.

Down:

1 - Covers the median nerve: **_FLEXOR_** retinaculum
For recalcitrant carpal tunnel syndrome, the retinaculum is cut to release the pressure on the nerve.

3 - Artery that runs through #13 down **_RADIAL_**

4 - One for the gunners: The ulnar nerve runs through this canal **_GUYON'S_**

5 - Damage to long **_THORACIC_** nerve can result in winged scapula
Might occur during a mastectomy.

6 - #21 down = **_CARPAL_** tunnel syndrome

9 - Foot drop can result from damage to common **_PERONEAL_** nerve

10 - Damaged **_RADIAL_** nerve could lead to wrist drop

12 - Damaged **_ULNAR_** nerve could lead to claw hand
Also known as Klumpke palsy.

13 - Area bordered by ligaments of extensor pollicis longus, extensor pollicis brevis, and abductor pollicis longus
SNUFFBOX

14 - The only one of the rotator cuff muscles that will fit in this spot of the puzzle
TERES MINOR. *Others are supraspinatus, infraspinatus, and subscapularis.*

16 - This wrist bone sits on the scaphoid and lunate
CAPITATE

17 - Tennis elbow = **_LATERAL_** epicondylitis
Classically presents with pain in elbow area with forearm activity like grasping or twisting. There is point tenderness over the lateral epicondyle.

18 - This wrist bone comes with a hook
HAMATE. *Hook of the hamate fracture might occur when you hit the ground hard with your golf club on the downswing; hamus is Latin for "hook."*

21 - Entrapment of **_MEDIAN_** nerve leads to paresthesias in thumb, index, and middle finger

16 A Puzzle to Earn Immunity

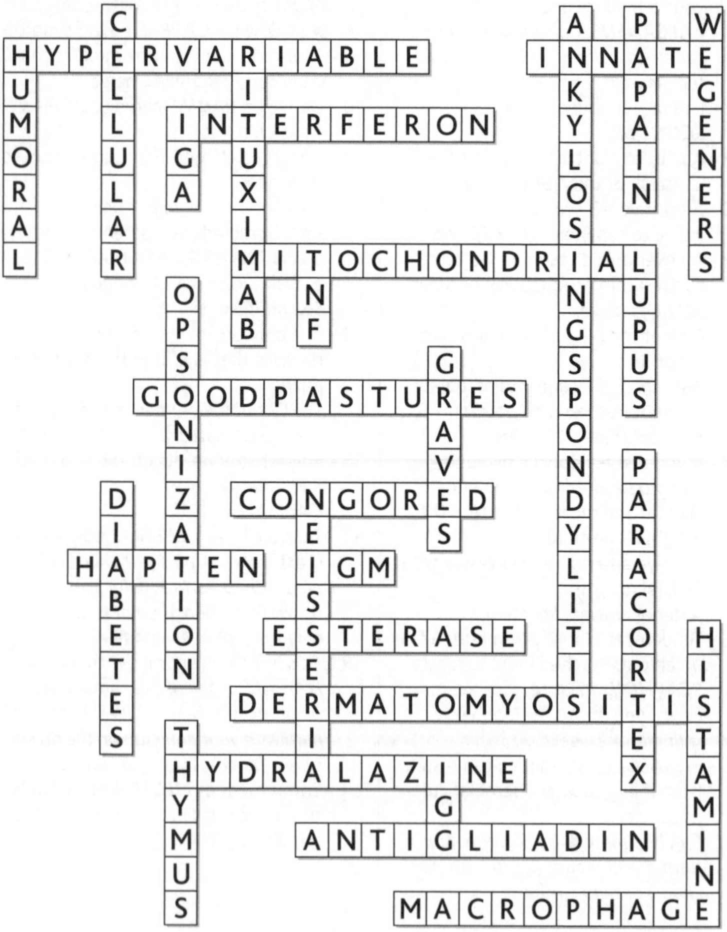
HYPERVARIABLE
INNATE
INTERFERON
MITOCHONDRIAL
GOODPASTURES
CONGORED
HAPTEN
IGM
ESTERASE
DERMATOMYOSITIS
HYDRALAZINE
ANTIGLIADIN
MACROPHAGE
CELLULAR
HUMORAL
RITUXIMAB
IGA
ANKYLOSINGSPONDYLITIS
PAPAIN
WEGENERS
TNF
OPSONIZATION
GRAVES
LUPUS
DIABETES
NEISSERI
PARACORTEX
HISTAMINE
THYMUS
IGG

Across:

5 - Determines antibody's antigen specificity: **HYPERVARIABLE** region

7 - Macrophages, neutrophils, and natural killer cells are part of our **INNATE** immunity
Those cells are natural born killers (but unfortunately have no memory).

8 - CD4+ T-cells make gamma-**INTERFERON**
This stuff activates macrophages.

9 - Primary biliary cirrhosis: Anti**MITOCHONDRIAL** antibodies

14 - Antibody to basement membrane: **GOODPASTURE'S** syndrome

17 - Stain used to spot amyloid (two words) **CONGO RED**

19 - Small molecule that can be antigenic when attached to a carrier **HAPTEN**

20 - First class of immunoglobulin produced upon antigenic exposure
IgM. *IgM is for our iMmediate immunity.*

21 - Hereditary angioedema is caused by the deficiency of C1 **ESTERASE** inhibitor

23 - Autoimmune connective tissue disorder characterized by heliotrope rash **DERMATOMYOSITIS**

25 - Vasodilator that can cause a lupus-like syndrome **HYDRALAZINE**

27 - Check these antibodies if you suspect celiac sprue
ANTIGLIADIN. *Also check antiendomysial.*

28 - This type of cell has major histocompatibility complex issues! Class II that is **MACROPHAGE**

Down:

1 - Live attenuated vaccines induce this type of active immune response
CELLULAR. *Inactivated or killed vaccines induce humoral response.*

2 - HLA-B27 disease (two words) **ANKYLOSING SPONDYLITIS**

3 - Two Fab fragments and an Fc results when this "does its thing" on an immunoglobulin **PAPAIN**

4 - c-ANCA: **WEGENER'S** granulomatosis

5 - B lymphocytes are major cells of the **HUMORAL** immune response
(It's not really funny.)

6 - Therapy used for non-Hodgkin lymphoma, it is an antibody to CD20 **RITUXIMAB**

8 - Immunoglobulin in breast milk
IgA. *Breastmilk – it does a baby body good.*

10 - Mediates septic shock: **TNF**-alpha (initials)
Tumor necrosis factor recruits white cells and activates the endothelium causing vasodilation and vascular "leakiness."

11 - Anti-dsDNA and anti-Smith, think **LUPUS** (short form)

12 - Fancy word for binding bacteria done by C3b
OPSONIZATION. *See if you can work this word in at your next dinner party.*

13 - Antibodies to the thyroid-stimulating hormone receptor: **GRAVES** disease
Very common thyroid disorder.

15 - Part of the lymph node that is home to Mr. T cells
PARACORTEX. *To paraphrase Mr. T: "I pity the fool ...who doesn't know his paracortex from his medulla."*

16 - HLA-DR3: Type 1 **DIABETES**

18 - Problems with complement pathway C5b to C9 may lead to recurrent infections by this genus **NEISSERIA**

22 - IgE causes its release from mast cells and basophils
HISTAMINE. *Elevated in patients with allergies and asthma; hypersensitive-"E" immunoglobulin.*

24 - A 22q11 deletion leads to failure of this to develop, leading to recurrent viral infections
THYMUS. *Infections due to T-cell deficiency; also known as DiGeorge syndrome, other effects are hypocalcemia (due to the absence of parathyroids) and congenital heart defects.*

26 - Most abundant type of immunoglobulin
IgG. *Responsible for lonG term immunity.*

17 Bug Hunt

Notes

18 For Old Timers' Sake

Meredith Gilliam

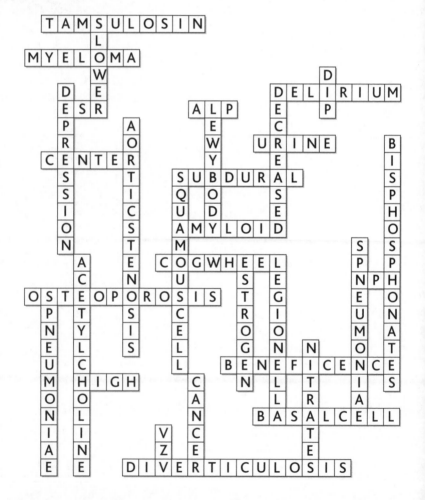

Across:

1 - An alpha-1 antagonist used in the treatment of benign prostatic hypertrophy
TAMSULOSIN

3 - Most likely diagnosis in an elderly person presenting with a pathologic fracture and "punched-out" lytic bone lesions on plain films: Multiple **MYELOMA**

6 - Term that describes acute onset waxing and waning level of consciousness in your elderly patient
DELIRIUM. Always search for underlying cause.

7 - Laboratory value (acronym) classically elevated in elderly woman with unilateral headache and vision loss
ESR. Temporal arteritis (giant cell arteritis) involves focal granulomatous inflammation of medium-large arteries, especially branches of the carotid.

8 - Osteitis deformans (Paget's disease), which is more common in older adults, is characterized by normal calcium, phosphate, and PTH, but increased **ALP** (acronym)
Alkaline phosphatase. Paget's disease of bone leads to abnormal bone architecture; classic findings include increased hat size and hearing loss from auditory foramen narrowing.

11 - To confirm the diagnosis in #20 down, you collect sputum and **URINE** for testing
Urine antigen testing for Legionella may confirm the diagnosis.

13 - Age-related macular degeneration is most likely to present with vision loss in this part of the visual field
CENTER. An area of central vision loss is called a scotoma.

14 - An elderly patient who fell 2 weeks ago and has progressive confusion might have this finding on a CT of his head: **SUBDURAL** hematoma
It is crescent-shaped versus epidural which is lens shaped.

15 - Senile plaques seen on brain microscopy in Alzheimer's disease comprises this type of protein
AMYLOID. Histologic findings in Alzheimer's disease include senile plaques (amyloid protein) and neurofibrillary tangles (intracellular, abnormally phosphorylated tau protein).

18 - Parkinson's disease is associated with this type of rigidity in the arms
COGWHEEL. The classic symptoms of Parkinson's disease are resting Tremor, cogwheel Rigidity, Akinesia, and Postural instability (mnemonic: A person with Parkinson's disease is TRAPped in her body).

21 - The diagnosis suggested by progressive dementia, ataxia, and urinary incontinence in an elderly woman (acronym)
NPH (normal pressure hydrocephalus). You may know the symptoms better as "weird, wobbly, and wet."

22 - The underlying diagnosis you should suspect in a thin elderly woman presenting with loss of height and kyphosis
OSTEOPOROSIS

25 - An elderly woman with advanced dementia lacks decision-making capacity. Her physician, acting in the patient's best interest, decides to admit her to a skilled nursing facility. What is the ethical principle guiding this physician's action?
BENEFICENCE. Refers to a physician's ethical duty to act in a patient's best interest; this principle may sometimes be at odds with the principle of patient autonomy.

26 - Presbycusis causes loss of **HIGH** frequency sounds first
Presbycusis results primarily from cochlear hair cell dysfunction, and falls in the sensorineural hearing loss category; also anything "presby-" (e.g., presbyopia) is associated with aging.

28 - This type of skin carcinoma, common in the elderly, is characterized by rolled edges with central ulceration (two words)
BASAL CELL. Pearly papules and telangectasias are also associated with basal cell carcinomas.

30 - This common condition in older adults is associated with low-fiber diets and increased intraluminal pressure in the distal colon
DIVERTICULOSIS. Mostly affects the sigmoid colon; inflammation/infection of diverticuli is called diverticulitis.

Down:

2 - Age-related changes may lead to (faster/slower) clearance of fat-soluble drugs
SLOWER. Due to increasing % body fat with age.

4 - Unlike rheumatoid arthritis, osteoarthritis may affect the **DIP** joints in the hands (acronym)
Degeneration of the DIP and PIP joints in osteoarthritis are known as Heberden's nodes and Bouchard's nodes, respectively.

5 - This condition may present in elderly patients as "pseudodementia"
DEPRESSION

6 - Unlike depression, aging is associated with (increased/decreased) REM sleep
DECREASED

9 - Most likely type of dementia in an elderly patient with rigidity, tremor, and hallucinations (two words)
LEWY BODY. Core clinical features of Lewy body dementia include cognitive fluctuations, visual hallucinations, and parkinsonism.

10 - This cardiac valve problem, prevalent in 2% to 9% of adults over 65, causes weak and late peripheral pulses (two words)
AORTIC STENOSIS. The weak and late pulses are called pulsus parvus et tardus.

12 - This class of drugs is a common first-line treatment for osteoporosis
BISPHOSPHONATES. Bisphosphonates usually end in the suffix -dronate; they inhibit osteoclast activity.

14 - Keratin pearls on the histopathology of a skin lesion in an older adult suggests this type of carcinoma (two words)
SQUAMOUS CELL. Squamous cell carcinomas present as ulcerative, red lesions, and may be associated with chronic draining sinuses.

16 - The most common cause of meningitis in the 60+ age group (shorten the genus to an initial)
SPNEUMONIAE

17 - Synthesis of this neurotransmitter may be reduced in Alzheimer's disease
ACETYLCHOLINE

19 - Age-related deficiency of this hormone is the cause of atrophic vaginitis
ESTROGEN. Atrophic vaginitis may cause itching, dyspareunia, and bleeding after intercourse; always rule out cancer as the cause of vaginal bleeding in a postmenopausal woman.

20 - The organism on the top of your differential when a tour group of octogenarians visiting a whirlpool spa, all get pneumonia (genus)
LEGIONELLA. Legionnaires' disease (caused by Legionella pneumophila) is transmitted by aerosolized water droplets.

23 - The most common cause of community-acquired pneumonia in the elderly (shorten the genus to an initial)
SPNEUMONIAE. Yep, there are two Strep pneumo answers in this puzzle.

24 - To avoid life-threatening hypotension, ask your elderly male patients if they are taking this class of medication before prescribing treatment for erectile dysfunction
NITRATES. cGMP phosphodiesterase inhibitors (sildenafil, other -afils) are contraindicated in patients taking nitrates.

27 - After heart disease, the second leading cause of death in adults >65 years old
CANCER. Cerebrovascular accident is the third leading cause according to this breakdown

29 - Vaccination against this virus in >60 years of age group decreases the likelihood of a painful rash (acronym)
VZV. Shingles is caused by reactivated varicella zoster virus.

19 Name that Drug!

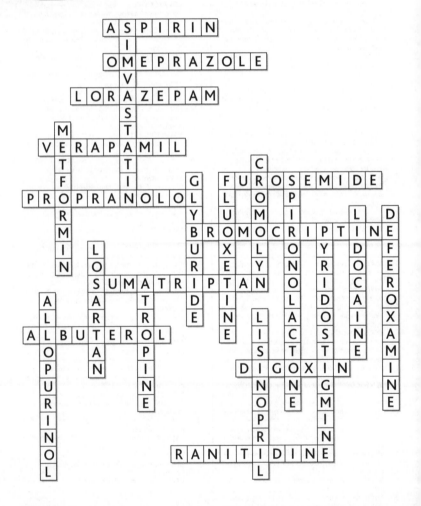

Across:

1 - Nonselectively and irreversibly inhibits cyclooxygenase
   ASPIRIN

3 - Inhibits gastric parietal cell H+K+ ATPase
   OMEPRAZOLE. *Proton pump inhibitors.*

4 - Binds to GABA receptors
   LORAZEPAM. *Benzodiazepines.*

6 - Nondihydropyridine blocker of calcium channels
   VERAPAMIL. *Diltiazem is another.*

9 - Inhibits loop of Henle sodium and chloride resorption
   FUROSEMIDE. *Loop diruretics.*

11 - Nonselectively antagonizes beta-1 and beta-2 adrenergic receptors
   PROPRANOLOL. *Nonselective beta-blockers.*

14 - Stimulates dopamine receptors
   BROMOCRIPTINE

17 - Used in migraine, this activates vascular serotonin 5-HT1 receptors
   SUMATRIPTAN. *Triptans.*

21 - Relaxes airways by selectively stimulating beta-2 adrenergic receptors
   ALBUTEROL. *B2-agonists.*

22 - Inhibits sodium–potassium ATPase
   DIGOXIN

23 - Selectively antagonizes H2 receptors
   RANITIDINE. *H2-blockers.*

Down:

2 - Inhibits 3-hydroxy-3-methylglutaryl-coenzyme A reductase
   SIMVASTATIN. *Statins.*

5 - Decreases hepatic glucose production, increases insulin sensitivity
   METFORMIN

7 - Inhibits mast cell degranulation
   CROMOLYN

8 - Stimulates pancreatic islet beta cell insulin release
   GLYBURIDE. *Sulfonylureas.*

9 - Selectively inhibits serotonin reuptake
   FLUOXETINE. *SSRIs.*

10 - Antagonizes distal convoluted tubule aldosterone receptors
   SPIRONOLACTONE

12 - Amide local anesthetic that inhibits Na ion channels
   LIDOCAINE

13 - Chelates iron
   DEFEROXAMINE

15 - Reversibly binds and inactivates acetylcholinesterase
   PYRIDOSTIGMINE

16 - Selectively antagonizes angiotensin II AT1 receptors
   LOSARTAN. *ARBs.*

18 - Antagonizes acetylcholine receptors
   ATROPINE

19 - Inhibits xanthine oxidase
   ALLOPURINOL

20 - Inhibits angiotensin-converting enzyme
   LISINOPRIL. *ACE inhibitors.*

20 Axis II

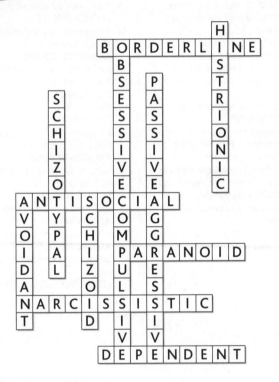

Across:

2 - Cluster B: Unstable, impulsive, vulnerable to abandonment, splitter **BORDERLINE**. *Glenn Close's character in Fatal Attraction.*

6 - Cluster B: Cannot conform to societal rules; criminal behavior **ANTISOCIAL**

8 - Cluster A: Mistrustful, hostile, suspicious, conspiracy theorist **PARANOID**

9 - Cluster B: Grandiose, overly sensitive to criticism, shows little empathy **NARCISSISTIC**

10 - Cluster C: Insecure, uncomfortable with decision-making or authority **DEPENDENT**

Down:

1 - Cluster B: Overemotional and dramatic **HISTRIONIC**. *Borderline can also be this way of course.*

3 - Cluster C: The stubborn perfectionist who likes all the soup cans lined up perfectly (two words) **OBSESSIVECOMPULSIVE**. *TV's Monk has OCD.*

4 - Cluster C: Noncompliant, procrastinator (two words) **PASSIVEAGGRESSIVE**

5 - Cluster A: Odd behaviors and thoughts but no psychosis **SCHIZOTYPAL**

6 - Cluster C: Involuntarily withdrawn and shy because fears rejection **AVOIDANT**

7 - Cluster A: Purposefully socially withdrawn, content living alone with no friends **SCHIZOID**

21 Kidney Klues

Yemeng Lu

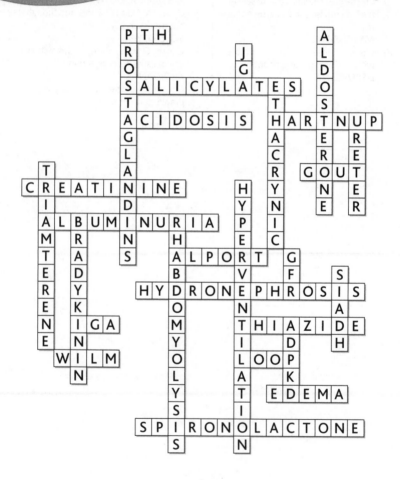

Across:

1 - **_PTH_** acts on the kidney to decrease renal phosphate reabsorption (acronym)
It is the major hormonal determinant of serum phosphate concentrations.

4 - "S" in MUDPILES for causes of increased anion gap
SALICYLATES. *MUDPILES: methanol, uremia, DKA, paraldehyde/phenformin, infection/iron/INH, lactic acidosis, ethylene glycol, salicylates.*

6 - pH abnormality that leads to hyperkalemia
ACIDOSIS. *It causes hyperkalemia by a shift of potassium out of cells.*

7 - Manifestation of deficiency of niacin/B3 can resemble **_HARTNUP_** disease
Autosomal recessive disorder caused by defective transport of neutral amino acids in the small intestine and the kidneys; patients present with pellagra-like symptoms.

10 - A patient loves to eat red meat, fatty seafood, and malt whiskey; he gets a kidney stone that is not visible on x-ray; he most likely also has **_GOUT_**
Uric acid kidney stones are radiolucent and strongly associated with conditions of hyperuricemia such as gout.

11 - **_CREATININE_** is moderately secreted by the renal tubules; therefore, it overestimates GFR

13 - A key feature of nephrotic syndrome
ALBUMINURIA

16 - Patient with bilateral hearing loss and microscopic hematuria may have **_ALPORT_** syndrome

19 - Your 65-year-old male patient takes 10 minutes to urinate, has a stop-and-go urine stream and still dribbles urine all day; progression of his condition can lead to **_HYDRONEPHROSIS_** of the kidneys
It results from urinary tract obstruction and leads to dilation up to the obstruction.

20 - **_IgA_** nephropathy is the most common lesion found to cause primary glomerulonephritis throughout most developed countries

21 - Early distal convoluted tubule is the site of action for these diuretics
THIAZIDE

23 - Most common renal malignancy in young children: **_WILM_**'s tumor

24 - Class of drugs that inhibits the $Na^+/2Cl^-/K^+$ symporters in the thick ascending limb of the nephron: **_LOOP_** diuretics

25 - A 6-year-old 2 weeks after a strep throat-infection with acute poststreptococcal glomerulonephritis will most likely present with **_EDEMA_**
Generalized edema is present in about two-thirds of patients due to sodium and water retention.

26 - Diuretic that can also be used for unfortunate ladies with excess body hair and do not enjoy a 5-o' clock shadow
SPIRONOLACTONE. *It has antiandrogen properties.*

Down:

1 - A woman with severe dysmenorrhea taking OTC pain medicines ends up with acute renal failure because of the inhibition of production of **_PROSTAGLANDINS_**
They keep the afferent arterioles vasodilated to maintain GFR.

2 - In the collecting tubules, this leads to insertion of Na^+ channel on the luminal side of the tubule
ALDOSTERONE

3 - Consists of modified smooth muscle cells, and Na^+ sensoring cells (acronym)
JGA. *It consists of the juxtaglomerular cells, the macula densa, and the lacis cells or agranular cells.*

5 - A patient with heart failure needs immediate medical diuresis but has a sulfa allergy; you use **_ETHACRYNIC_** acid and save the day
It has no cross-reactivity to sulfonamides or sulfonylureas, while loop diuretics do.

8 - "Water under the bridge" = **_URETER_** passes under the uterine artery

9 - A potassium-sparing diuretic
TRIAMTERENE. *Spironolactone is another.*

12 - Compensatory response to metabolic acidosis
HYPERVENTILATION. *It will blow off more CO_2 and therefore increase pH.*

14 - Angiotensin II receptor blockers are less associated with cough compared to ACE inhibitors because they do not increase **_BRADYKININ_**

15 - Patient's leg was crushed in a high speed MVA and later developed acute tubular necrosis; the mechanism is **_RHABDOMYOLYSIS_**
It can lead to extreme enzyme elevations, electrolyte imbalances, and acute kidney injury.

17 - Inulin is neither secreted nor reabsorbed, thus can be used to approximate **_GFR_** (acronym)

18 - Hyponatremia, hypoosmolality, high urine osmolality, and high urine sodium concentration point to **_SIADH_** (acronym)
Condition where water excretion is partially impaired because of the inability to suppress the secretion of ADH.

22 - CT scan of the patient reveals massively enlarged kidneys bilaterally; he has **_ADPKD_** (acronym)
Typical findings on imaging include large kidneys and extensive cysts scattered throughout both kidneys.

22 Clinical Scramble

CAREYONDS

S	E	C	O	N	D	A	R	Y

HARS

R	A	S	H

LIPSANES

P	A	I	N	L	E	S	S

HACCREN

C	H	A	N	C	R	E

SHOPTIRECE

S	P	I	R	O	C	H	E	T	E

DIAGNOSIS: _____ **SYPHILIS** _____

Notes

23 A Gravid Situation

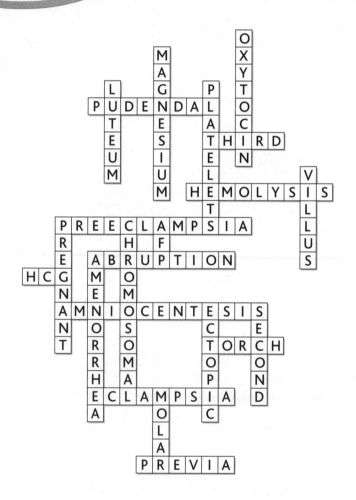

Across:

5 - Nerve block that can ease the pain of childbirth
PUDENDAL

6 - Stage of labor during which placenta is passed
THIRD. *Retained placental products can be a cause of postpartum hemorrhage.*

8 - The "H" in HELLP
HEMOLYSIS

9 - Hypertension and proteinuria during the second half of pregnancy
PREECLAMPSIA. *Definitive treatment is delivery.*

12 - Premature separation of placenta from uterine wall: Placental **ABRUPTION**
Painful bleeding in third trimester.

13 - Elevated in urine and blood if pregnant: Beta- **HCG** (acronym)
Human chorionic gonadotropin.

14 - Aspiration of fluid from the amniotic sac for purposes of analysis
AMNIOCENTESIS

17 - Classic acronym for infections that cause birth defects (Hint: Not the Olympic one)
TORCH. *Toxoplasmosis, Other (coxsackie, syphilis, varicella, HIV, parvovirus B19), Rubella, Cytomegalovirus, Herpes simplex virus.*

18 - #9 across with seizures
ECLAMPSIA. *Treatment for eclamptic seizure is IV magnesium.*

20 - Placenta blocking the cervix: Placenta **PREVIA**
Painless vaginal bleeding. Do not perform a digital cervical exam until you make sure that it is NOT a previa.

Down:

1 - Hormone that stimulates contractions
OXYTOCIN

2 - Intravenous treatment for preeclampsia while waiting for delivery
MAGNESIUM

3 - Produces progesterone and estrogen during the first trimester: Corpus **LUTEUM**

4 - The "P" in HELLP
PLATELETS. *The preceding L is for Low.*

7 - Can be performed earlier than #14 across, if needed, to evaluate for genetic abnormalities: Chorionic **VILLUS** sampling

9 - Clinically, assume all women of childbearing age are this until you have evidence to the contrary
PREGNANT. *Evidence can be history of hysterectomy, known LMP, or a pregnancy test when needed.*

10 - Most common cause of miscarriage: **CHROMOSOMAL** abnormalities

11 - One of the substances measured to screen for neural tube defects (acronym)
AFP. *Alpha-fetoprotein.*

12 - Absence of menses
AMENORRHEA

15 - Implantation outside the uterine cavity: **ECTOPIC** pregnancy
An emergency not to miss! Think of ectopic in any woman of childbearing age with abdominal or pelvic pain.

16 - Stage of labor from complete dilation until birth (the "pushing" stage)
SECOND

19 - "Snowstorm" on ultrasound; cluster of grapes on pathology specimen: **MOLAR** pregnancy
AKA hydatidiform mole.

24 Doc, There's a Worm in My...

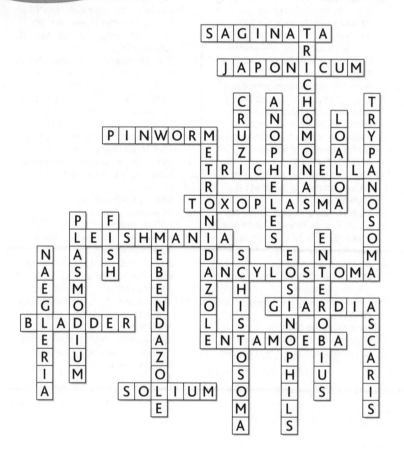

Across:

1 - Beef tapeworm species
   SAGINATA
3 - Schistosoma species whose egg has a lateral spine
   JAPONICUM
8 - Scotch tape test used to diagnose this infection (common name)
   PINWORM. *Patients often have anal itching.*
10 - Eating undercooked meat may lead to infection with this (genus), which has the double-barreled egg
   TRICHINELLA
11 - Pregnant women should not clean the kitty litter because of possibility of infection with this (genus)
   TOXOPLASMA
14 - Kala-azar is the visceral form of the infection caused by this genus
   LEISHMANIA
20 - Causes cutaneous larvae migrans (genus)
   ANCYLOSTOMA
21 - Flagellated protozoan that causes diarrhea (genus)
   GIARDIA
23 - *Schistosoma haematobium* might infect this if you are peeing in a river in Egypt
   BLADDER
24 - Can cause liver abscess: **ENTAMOEBA** histolytica
   The classic is anchovy paste liver abscess.
25 - Pork tapeworm species
   SOLIUM

Down:

2 - Causes vaginitis/cervicitis with "strawberry cervix" (genus)
   TRICHOMONAS.
4 - Chagas disease is caused by trypanosoma **CRUZI** (species)
5 - Kind of female mosquito that transmits malaria
   ANOPHELES
6 - Causes sleeping sickness: **TRYPANOSOMA** brucei
7 - Double-sounding eye worm disease
   LOALOA
9 - Treatment for #2 down
   METRONIDAZOLE
12 - Malaria genus
   PLASMODIUM
13 - *Diphyllobothrium latum* is the **FISH** tapeworm
15 - Antiparasitic used for many worm infections
   MEBENDAZOLE
16 - Pinworm (genus)
   ENTEROBIUS
17 - "Brain-eating ameba" from warm freshwater up the nose (genus)
   NAEGLERIA (FOWLERI)
18 - Blood fluke (genus)
   SCHISTOSOMA
19 - These kinds of white blood cells are often elevated in parasitic infection
   EOSINOPHILS
22 - These roundworms can cause an intestinal blockage (genus)
   ASCARIS

25 Catching My Breath

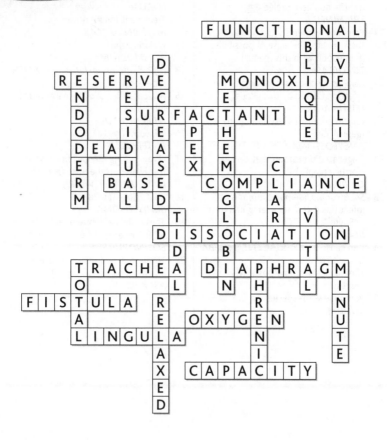

Across:

1 - # 7 down + ERV = **FUNCTIONAL** residual capacity

5 - After you take a normal breath in, the extra volume you can breathe in: Inspiratory **RESERVE** volume
Similarly, there is an expiratory reserve volume beyond the tidal volume.

8 - Carbon **MONOXIDE** has about 200 times the affinity for hemoglobin than O_2
This will cause a left shift in the curve and decrease O_2 unloading to the tissues.

9 - Type II pneumocytes produce this important stuff
SURFACTANT

11 - Part of the respiratory tree where no gas exchange takes place: The **DEAD** space

13 - This portion of the lung has some wasted perfusion
BASE

14 - The change in lung volume for a given change in pressure is termed
COMPLIANCE

17 - No doubt, one of your favorite things: The oxygen–hemoglobin **DISSOCIA-TION** curve

18 - Bifurcation of this occurs at around T5
TRACHEA

19 - C3, C4, and C5 keep this alive
DIAPHRAGM. *These roots form the phrenic nerve.*

22 - If the lung bud does not completely separate from the esophagus, a tracheoesophageal **FISTULA** forms

24 - "A summary of medicine: Air goes in and out, blood goes round and round, and **OXYGEN** is good"
Well, maybe there is a bit more to it...

25 - The left lung has no middle lobe but has this
LINGULA

26 - #5 across + #15 down = inspiratory
CAPACITY
Remember that when you add any two or more lung volumes together, you get a capacity.

Down:

2 - Separates right middle lobe from right inferior lobe: **OBLIQUE** fissure

3 - Most of these air sacs actually do not develop until after we are born
ALVEOLI

4 - When #17 across shifts to the right, there is (increased/decreased) affinity for O_2
DECREASED

6 - The lining of the respiratory tract is derived from this embryonic layer
ENDODERM. *Muscle layer and connective tissue come from mesoderm.*

7 - Volume that stays in the lungs after maximal expiration
RESIDUAL. *This cannot be measured by spirometry.*

8 - Oxidized form of hemoglobin
METHEMOGLOBIN. *Does not bind O_2 well.*

10 - This portion of the lung has some wasted ventilation
APEX

12 - Nonciliated cells with secretory granules: **CLARA** cells

15 - The volume expired with a normal breath: **TIDAL** volume
This is typically about 500 mL.

16 - #5 across + #15 down + ERV = **VITAL** capacity

18 - #5 across + #15 down + #7 down + ERV = **TOTAL** lung capacity

20 - Provides the electrical "juice" to the diaphragm: **PHRENIC** nerve

21 - **MINUTE** ventilation = TV × respiratory rate

23 - This form of hemoglobin is really ready to bind some O_2
RELAXED. *The taut form is too uptight to bind it.*

26 Just for Fun: I'm not a Doctor...*

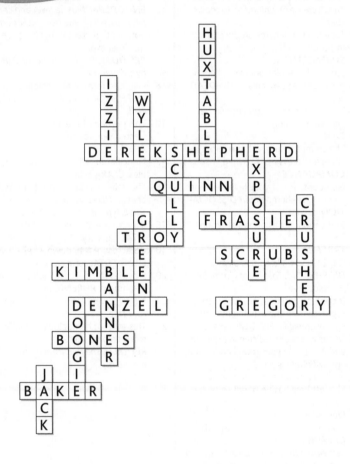

*... but I play one on TV

Across:

4 - Dr. McDreamy's real (well, still fake) name (first and last) **DEREKSHEPHERD**. *Played by Patrick Dempsey (who played a nerd in many of his 80s movies).*

7 - Dr. **QUINN**: Medicine Woman

10 - Psychiatrist frequently seen at the bar in Cheers: Dr. **FRASIER** Crane *Actually had his own spinoff.*

11 - Narcissistic plastic surgeon on Nip/Tuck: Dr. Christian **TROY**

12 - Dr. Kim Briggs, Dr. Molly Clock, Dr. Walter Mickhead, Dr. Grace Miller: Some characters on **SCRUBS**

13 - The Fugitive (was also a movie): Dr. Richard **KIMBLE** *Vascular surgeon.*

15 - Got his start acting as a doctor on St. Elsewhere: **DENZEL** Washington *Check out that hair.*

16 - House's first name (in the show) **GREGORY**

17 - Nickname of Dr. Leonard McCoy on the original Star Trek **BONES**. *Dammit Jim, I'm a doctor!*

19 - Little House on the Prairie's doc: Dr. **BAKER** *A great simple country doc, he also was the town veterinarian.*

Down:

1 - Dr. Heathcliff **HUXTABLE** in the Cosby Show *Obstetrician and great family man.*

2 - Dr. **IZZIE** Stevens (nickname) played by Katherine Heigl

3 - Played Carter on ER: Noah **WYLE** *Did you know he was in the movie A Few Good Men?*

5 - One of the two investigators on the X-Files: Dr. Dana **SCULLY** *Her partner was Fox Mulder.*

6 - Dr. Joel Fleischman: Northern **EXPO-SURE**

8 - STNG (for the non-Trekkies, that's Star Trek: The Next Generation) doctor Beverly **CRUSHER**

9 - Anthony Edwards' character on ER: Dr. Mark **GREENE**

14 - Turned into the Incredible Hulk: Dr. David **BANNER** *Physician and scientist; In the comics, he went by Bruce.*

15 - **DOOGIE** Howser, MD *Somehow they got around that age requirement for a medical license.*

18 - Matthew Fox played Dr. **JACK** Shephard on Lost *He was a neurosurgeon. His tattoos are real.*

27 Codons on Coffee Break

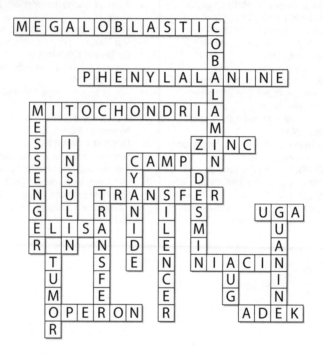

Across:

1 - Deficiency of #2 down causes this type of anemia
MEGALOBLASTIC. *Can lead to neuropathy also.*

3 - An essential amino acid; this one is found in many diet sodas
PHENYLALANINE

4 - Cellular site of oxidative phosphorylation (plural)
MITOCHONDRIA

6 - Element essential for the function of multitude of enzymes. Some say it helps the common cold.
ZINC. *Not sure whether it really works.*

7 - A second messenger increased by the activation of a type of G protein
CAMP. *Cyclic adenosine monophosphate.*

9 - This RNA reads the code
TRANSFER

11 - STOP! In the name of this codon (not UAA or UAG)
UGA

13 - Laboratory technique in which antigen–antibody reactivity is tested (acronym)
ELISA. *Enzyme-linked immunosorbent assay.*

15 - Pellagra is caused by the deficiency of this B vitamin
NIACIN. *Pellagra patients can have the four Ds: Diarrhea, dermatitis, dementia, and death*

17 - This genetic structure regulates transcription
OPERON

18 - The fat-soluble vitamins (alphabetical order)
ADEK

Down:

2 - Fancier name for vitamin B12
COBALAMIN. *If deficient, can be given intramuscularly or orally, contrary to popular belief.*

4 - The longest type of RNA
MESSENGER

5 - This hormone can be thought of as our storage stimulator
INSULIN

7 - This toxin directly blocks electron flow through the electron transport chain
CYANIDE

8 - Muscle cells can be immunochemically stained using this protein
DESMIN

9 - RNA that carries amino acids
TRANSFER

10 - Genetic site at which negative regulators bind (also might be seen being used in a different capacity in mafia movies)
SILENCER

12 - One of the purines (would not "The Purines" be a great band name?)
GUANINE. *Adenosine is the other.*

14 - p53 is a _____ suppressor protein
TUMOR

16 - "Let's Get it Started (in Here)" by the Black Eyed Peas might be this codon's theme song
AUG

28 Achy Breaky Heart

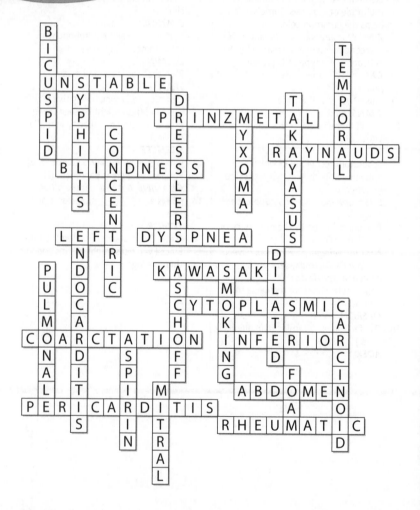

Across:

3 - Cardiac chest pain at rest or escalating in severity = **_UNSTABLE_** angina
Note that unstable angina is a clinical diagnosis. ECG and cardiac enzymes may be normal.

7 - Coronary vasospasm = **_PRINZMETAL_** angina

10 - Vasospasm in the fingers and toes in response to cold temperature or stress **_RAYNAUD'S_**. *Can be seen with connective tissue diseases, but can also be isolated.*

11 - The worrisome sequela of #2 down **_BLINDNESS_**. *High-dose steroids are given to prevent blindness.*

12 - Most common cause of right heart failure: **_LEFT_** heart failure

14 - **_DYSPNEA_** on exertion is a cardinal symptom of congestive heart failure
Due to the inability of cardiac output to increase during exercise.

17 - Coronary artery aneurysms may be seen as a complication of this syndrome that affects young children: **_KAWASAKI_** disease
Typical board examination patient is a 5-year-old Asian girl with fever, swollen lymph nodes, red eyes/lips, and desquamation of the finger tips. Treatment is IV immunoglobulin and aspirin.

20 - Antineutrophil **_CYTOPLASMIC_** antibody
ANCA can be associated with vasculitis.

22 - Absent femoral pulses on examination, hypertension (in arms), and rib notching: **_COARCTATION_** of the aorta
More common in boys.

24 - Q waves on ECG in leads II, III, and aVF suggest a prior MI along the **_INFERIOR_** wall
V1 – V4 = anterior; V1 – V2 = anteroseptal.

27 - Most common site for an aortic aneurysm **_ABDOMEN_**. *Older male smokers/ex-smokers are the most common risk group for AAA.*

28 - Diffuse, upwardly concave ST segment elevation on ECG: Acute **_PERICARDITIS_**

29 - Anitschkow cells, previous strep throat, mitral valve stenosis: **_RHEUMATIC_** fever
Note that rheumatic heart disease is immune mediated (antibodies to M protein), not directly due to the bacteria.

Down:

1 - This congenital heart defect is associated with aortic stenosis: **_BICUSPID_** aortic valve

2 - Elderly woman with unilateral headache and jaw pain, might also have stiffness in shoulders: **_TEMPORAL_** arteritis
Associated with polymyalgia rheumatica. ESR is typically very high.

4 - Ascending aortic aneurysm may be a result of this infection
SYPHILIS

5 - Autoimmune pericarditis that can follow a myocardial infarction: **_DRESSLER'S_** syndrome
Happens several weeks after an MI.

6 - "Pulseless disease": **_TAKAYASU'S_** arteritis
Due to granulomatous thickening of aortic arch, leading to weak upper extremity pulses.

8 - Most common primary cardiac neoplasm in adults: Atrial **_MYXOMA_**
These are usually left-sided.

9 - Heart's response to chronic hypertension = **_CONCENTRIC_** hypertrophy of the left ventricle

13 - Splinter hemorrhages, on examination, in patient with fever: Think **_ENDOCARDITIS_**
Other signs include Roth spots, Janeway lesions, Osler's nodes, and murmur.

15 - Most common type of cardiomyopathy **_DILATED_**. *Also called "congestive," represents about 90% of the cases.*

16 - Cause of isolated right heart failure: Cor **_PULMONALE_**

18 - Foci of collagen surrounded by lymphocytes and macrophages pathognomonic for rheumatic heart disease: **_ASCHOFF_** bodies
The macrophages in this case are called Anitschkow cells

19 - Thromboangiitis obliterans (Buerger's disease) is due to **_SMOKING_**

21 - If a patient has stenosis of a right-sided heart valve, consider this syndrome **_CARCINOID_**. *Other clinical findings may include flushing, GI hypermotility, broncho-constriction, and hepatomegaly.*

23 - Antiplatelet drug used for primary and secondary prevention of coronary artery disease
ASPIRIN

25 - Macrophages ingest oxidized LDL in the vessel wall to become **_FOAM_** cells

26 - Most frequently infected heart valve **_MITRAL_**

29 It's Raining MEN (and other Endocrine Pathologies)

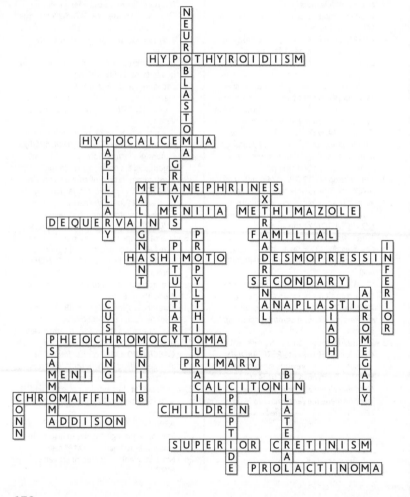

Across:

2 - Name the disease: Weight gain, constipation, dry skin, cold intolerance
HYPOTHYROIDISM

3 - Involuntary twitching of facial muscles, when facial nerve is tapped, occurs with this electrolyte abnormality
HYPOCALCEMIA. *This is called the Chvostek sign and is caused by tetanic contractions of the facial nerve.*

6 - Checking for these in the urine will clinch the diagnosis of pheochromocytoma
METANEPHRINES. *A diagnosis you might make once in your career.*

8 - It's Raining MEN: Medullary thyroid cancer, pheochromocytoma, hyperparathyroidism
MEN IIA. *Aka, Sipple Syndrome.*

9 - Antithyroid drug preferred in absence of pregnancy
METHIMAZOLE

10 - _____ thyroiditis: A transient hyperthyroid state, associated with a painful goiter, granulomatous inflammation of the thyroid
DEQUERVAIN('S). *Aka, subacute thyroiditis. Thought to be viral in origin. May occur postpartum.*

12 - Pheochromocytoma rule of 10s
FAMILIAL. *(Each of these "rule of 10s" answers applies to 10% of pheochromocytoma, a disease you will be taught and tested about over and over again, and never see.)*

15 - _____ thyroiditis: Most common cause of hypothyroidism in adults (eponym)
HASHIMOTO('S). *Also probably the most common autoimmune disease there is.*

16 - Drug used in the treatment of central diabetes insipidus
DESMOPRESSIN. *A vasopressin/ADH agonist.*

17 - Form of hyperparathyroidism associated with the chronic renal disease, hypocalcemia
SECONDARY. *Characterized by normal or hyperphosphatemia.*

20 - Worst thyroid carcinoma
ANAPLASTIC. *Five-year survival rate is between 5% and 10%.*

22 - Name the tumor: Paroxysmal hypertension, headache, hyperhidrosis, hyperthermia, hypermetabolism
PHEOCHROMOCYTOMA. *Manifestations all due to surge in catecholamines.*

24 - Form of hyperparathyroidism associated with excess PTH and hypercalcemia
PRIMARY. *Characterized by hypophosphatemia.*

25 - It's Raining MEN: Parathyroid hyperplasia, pancreatic islet cell tumors, pituitary tumors
MEN I. *Aka, Wermer Syndrome. Remember this one does NOT include pheo.*

27 - Medullary thyroid cancer secretes this hormone
CALCITONIN. *Produced by the C-cells in the thyroid.*

29 - These cells migrate from the neural crest and form adrenal medulla
CHROMAFFIN. *These are the cells that go awry in pheochromocytoma.*

30 - Pheochromocytoma rule of 10s
CHILDREN

31 - Name the disease: Hypotension, hyponatremia, hyperpigmentation
ADDISON('S). *Primary adrenal insufficiency. JFK had this disease.*

32 - Fourth pharyngeal pouch forms the superior/inferior parathyroid
SUPERIOR. *It's the opposite of what you'd think.*

33 - Common cause of mental retardation in the developing world
CRETINISM. *A form of hypothyroidism due to poor intake of iodine.*

34 - Name the tumor: Amenorrhea, galactorrhea
PROLACTINOMA. *Diagnosed by MRI definitively.*

Down:

1 - Name the tumor: Malignant abdominal mass in children, related to the N-myc oncogene
NEUROBLASTOMA

4 - Most common thyroid cancer, best prognosis
PAPILLARY

5 - Name the disease: Tachycardia, exophthalmos, weight loss
GRAVES

6 - Pheochromocytoma rule of 10s
MALIGNANT

7 - Pheochromocytoma rule of 10s
EXTRAADRENAL

11 - Antithyroid drug preferred for treating hyperthyroidism in pregnancy
PROPYLTHIOURACIL

13 - The Rathke's pouch forms the anterior lobe of this gland
PITUITARY. *Secretes FSH, LH, ACTH, TSH, prolactin, estrogen, GH.*

14 - Third pharyngeal pouch forms the superior/inferior parathyroid
INFERIOR. *It's the opposite of what you'd think.*

18 - Name the disease: Large hands and feet
ACROMEGALY. *Due to growth hormone excess.*

19 - Name the syndrome: Central obesity, moon facies, buffalo hump, abdominal striae
CUSHING('S). *Most commonly due to exogenous steroid administration.*

21 - Common cause of hyponatremia, seen in many diseases, classically small-cell lung cancer (acronym)
SIADH (SYNDROME OF INAPPROPRIATE ANTIDIURETIC HORMONE). *Just about any process that affects the lungs or CNS can cause this.*

22 - Histologic "body" may be seen in #4 down and a number of other cancers
PSAMMOMA. *Also seen in ovarian papillary serous adenocarcinoma, meningioma, gastric adenocarcinoma, and many others.*

23 - It's Raining MEN: Mucosal neuroma, medullary thyroid cancer, marfanoid, pheochromocytoma
MEN IIB. *Aka, MEN III. Both forms of MEN II are associated with mutations in the RET oncogene.*

26 - Pheochromocytoma rule of 10s
BILATERAL

28 - Levels of this byproduct of endogenous insulin production will be low in type I diabetes and high in type II diabetes
C-PEPTIDE

29 - Name the syndrome: Hypertension, hypokalemia, low renin level
CONN. *Aka, primary hyperaldosteronism.*

30 A Bug's Life 2

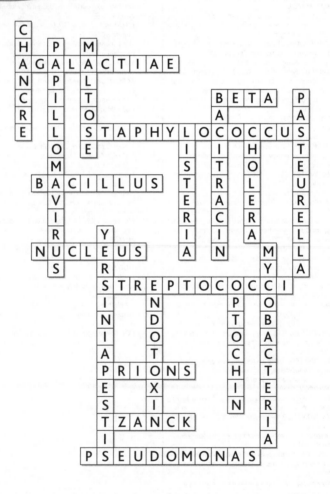

Across:

4 - Group B strep is also known as streptococcus ***AGALACTIAE*** (species)

5 - Group A strep are ***BETA***-hemolytic

7 - Catalase-positive, gram-positive cocci (genus)
STAPHYLOCOCCUS

10 - A spore-forming, gram-positive rod genus (think bad fried rice)
BACILLUS. *Bacillus cereus causes food poisoning (big-time vomiting and diarrhea); the classic story is from fried rice that was sitting out all day.*

12 - You will find most DNA viruses replicating here
NUCLEUS. *Poxvirus is an exception.*

14 - Gram-positive cocci in chains (genus)
STREPTOCOCCI. *I think of "strips" (sounds like "streps") being like chains.*

17 - They have no DNA or RNA, but can still cause an infection
PRIONS. *They are made up only of proteins. Remember not to eat bad brains.*

18 - Use this smear of a sample from an unroofed vesicle to test for herpes
TZANCK. *Classic memory aid is "Tzanck heavens I don't have herpes."*

19 - This lactose nonfermenting gram-negative rod is oxidase-positive (genus only)
PSEUDOMONAS. *These are nasty buggers; if you have a board question about a patient with cystic fibrosis who has an infection, think pseudomonas.*

Down:

1 - Primary syphilis presents with a painless ***CHANCRE***

2 - Double-stranded circular DNA virus that causes warts
PAPILLOMAVIRUS

3 - Neisseria meningitidis ferments this sugar
MALTOSE

5 - Group A strep are ***BACITRACIN***-sensitive (and this drug can be used topically for impetigo)

6 - A board question about cat bites should make you think of this organism (genus)
PASTEURELLA

8 - The only gram-positive with lipopolysaccharide-lipid A (genus)
LISTERIA

9 - The toxin from it causes severe watery diarrhea by overactivating adenylate cyclase
CHOLERA. *Disables a G protein, which leads to chloride secretion in gut.*

11 - The organism that causes plague (two words)
YERSINIA PESTIS

13 - Gram-positive and acid-fast (genus, plural)
MYCOBACTERIA. *Tuberculosis is caused by a mycobacterium.*

15 - Gram-negatives often contain this heat-stable lipopolysaccharide in their outer membrane (it makes people sick)
ENDOTOXIN. *Fever and shock through TNF and IL-1.*

16 - S. pneumoniae and S. viridans, both alpha-hemolytic, can be told apart because S. pneumoniae is ***OPTO-CHIN*** sensitive

31 Inheritance

Notes

32 My Neurotransmitters are Acting Up

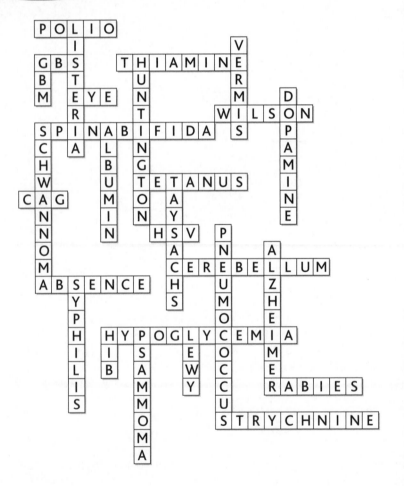

Across:

1 - Rarely seen paralysis from damage to LMNs caused by this virus
POLIO. *Thanks to vaccination, courtesy of Jonas Salk.*

4 - Most common cause of neonatal meningitis (acronym)
GBS (GROUP B STREPTOCOCCUS)

5 - Degeneration of mamillary bodies results from deficiency of this vitamin
THIAMINE. *Which may lead to Wernicke's encephalopathy seen in alcoholics. Always give thiamine before glucose to an alcoholic.*

7 - Location of the ring seen in #9 across
EYE. *The Kayser–Fleischer ring.*

9 - Liver disease which causes copper accumulation
WILSON('S). *Most common in young adults.*

10 - Most common neural tube defect (two words)
SPINA BIFIDA

12 - Neurotoxin that inhibits glycine release
TETANUS

14 - This trinucleotide repeat leads sufferers to "dance"
CAG. *Huntington's chorea ("choreia" is Greek for dance).*

15 - Xanthochromia and RBCs in the CSF should raise suspicion for this infection (acronym)
HSV (HERPES SIMPLEX VIRUS)

18 - Part of the brain most sensitive to alcohol
CEREBELLUM. *Hence the ataxic gait of a drunk.*

19 - Seizure of childhood characterized by blank stare
ABSENCE. *May be precipitated by having the child hyperventilate.*

21 - This metabolic abnormality may create a stroke mimic
HYPOGLYCEMIA. *Always check the glucose in any suspected stroke.*

24 - Negri bodies are seen in this uniformly fatal disease
RABIES. *Carried by bats and many wild rodents.*

25 - Neurotoxin that blocks glycine receptor
STRYCHNINE

Down:

2 - Bug that causes meningitis only in the very young or very old
LISTERIA. *Found in unpasteurized dairy products.*

3 - Arnold–Chiari malformation leads to herniation of this cerebellar structure
VERMIS

4 - Pseudopalisading arrangement of cells characterizes this devastating CNS tumor (acronym)
GBM (GLIOBLASTOMA MULTIFORME)

6 - Disease of #14 across
HUNTINGTON('S)

8 - Depletion of this neurotransmitter leads to a disorder characterized by a resting tremor
DOPAMINE

10 - Tumor often seen bilaterally in neurofibromatosis type 2
SCHWANNOMA. *Mutation on chromosome 22.*

11 - Guillain–Barre syndrome is a postviral ascending paralysis with high **ALBUMIN** levels in the CSF

13 - Deficiency in hexosaminidase A, cherry-red spot on macula
TAY-SACHS. *Common among Ashkenazi Jews.*

16 - Most common cause of meningitis in elderly (species form)
PNEUMOCOCCUS

17 - This most common form of dementia occurs at earlier age in individuals with trisomy 21
ALZHEIMER('S)

20 - Loss of touch, vibration, proprioception to the lower extremities caused by advanced form of this infection
SYPHILIS. *Also known as "tabes dorsalis," a manifestation of tertiary syphilis.*

21 - Cause of meningitis in children on the decline, thanks to this immunization (acronym)
HIB (HAEMOPHILUS INFLUENZAE B)

22 - Histologic features of meningioma: **PSAMMOMA** body (also seen in a variety of other tumors)
Also seen in ovarian papillary serous adenocarcinoma, papillary thyroid carcinoma, gastric adenocarcinoma, and many others.

23 - Type of "body" seen histologically in #8 down
LEWY. *Also seen in Lewy body dementia (think Alzheimer's + Parkinson's).*

33 GI Fizziology

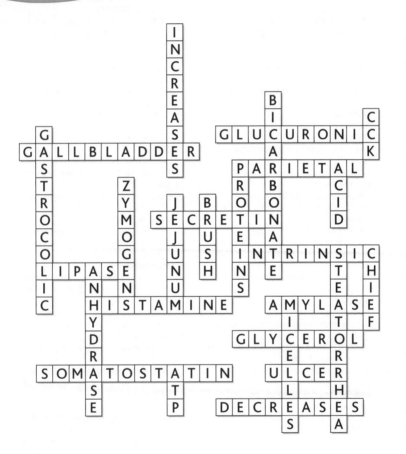

Across:

5 - Direct bilirubin is conjugated with this acid before being excreted in bile
GLUCURONIC

6 - CCK stimulates contraction of this (Useless hint: Not the uterus)
GALLBLADDER

7 - These cells secrete gastric acid
PARIETAL. *Important in acid reflux and ulcer pathophysiology.*

12 - Hormone that acts on the pancreatic ductal cells to increase mucus and bicarb secretion
SECRETIN

13 - Binds vitamin B12 for absorption in terminal ileum: **INTRINSIC** factor
Loss of intrinsic factor leads to B12 deficiency.

16 - Your pancreas probably secretes a lot of this after you eat at your favorite fast food restaurant
LIPASE. *Lipase helps digest fat; salivary glands also secrete some lipase.*

18 - Mast cells secrete this
HISTAMINE

19 - Secreted by salivary glands, this helps digest starches
AMYLASE. *Pancreas also secretes amylase.*

21 - Lipase turns triglycerides into fatty acids and this
GLYCEROL

22 - The D cells secrete this
SOMATOSTATIN

24 - If your patient has a tumor that is producing a lot of gastrin, a potential complication is this
ULCER

25 - If histamine is blocked, gastric acid (increases/decreases)
DECREASES. *This is how H2-blockers work.*

Down:

1 - If prostaglandin production is decreased, gastric acid (increases/decreases)
INCREASES. *This is why NSAIDs increase ulcer risk.*

2 - The presence of this in the stomach helps neutralize the acid
BICARBONATE

3 - The I cells of the duodenum and jejunum secrete this (acronym)
CCK. *Cholecystikinin.*

4 - My mom always says food goes "right through her"; what she does not understand is this reflex
GASTROCOLIC. *I have explained to my mom that the "food" coming out is not what she just ate.*

7 - Pepsinogen comes in handy to digest these
PROTEINS

8 - Acetylcholine stimulates production of this in the stomach
ACID

9 - CCK also stimulates the acinar cells of the pancreas to release these (Hint: The first letter is worth 10 points in Scrabble)
ZYMOGENS. *Zymogens are proenzymes (e.g., of the proteases).*

10 - Folate is absorbed in this part of the intestine
JEJUNUM

11 - Small intestine "border" that when wiped out can lead to diarrhea
BRUSH

14 - If your intestines are not absorbing fat properly (say, because your ileum is missing), you might develop "greasy stools"; this is called **STEATORRHEA**
You might have wanted to put "gross" but noticed that was not enough letters.

15 - These cells secrete pepsinogen
CHIEF

17 - Enzyme that turns CO_2 and H_2O into H^+ and HCO_3^-: Carbonic **ANHYDRASE**
This happens in the parietal cell.

20 - Long-chain fatty acids form these prior to passive diffusion
MICELLES

23 - The stomach's proton pump is an H^+/K^+ **ATP**ase pump

34 BMJ (Bones, Muscles, Joints)

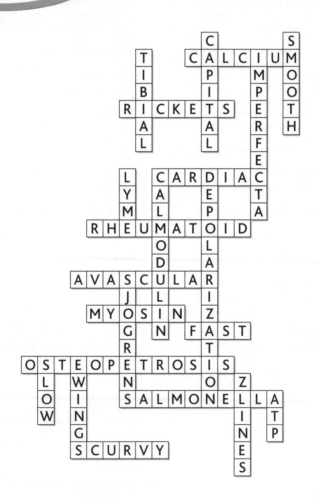

Across:

4 - Released from sarcoplasmic reticulum in response to #9 down
CALCIUM. *Calcium binds troponin C, causing it to undergo transformational change.*

6 - Disease of poor calcification of bone leading to bowing of legs in children
RICKETS. *Due to vitamin D deficiency.*

8 - If you were one of these kinds of muscle fibers your disks would be intercalated
CARDIAC

10 - Pannus formation in joints = **RHEU-MATOID** arthritis
It's autoimmune.

11 - Legg–Calve–Perthes disease is **AVAS-CULAR** necrosis of the head of the femur
Typically presents as painless limp in obese adolescent.

13 - Actin and **MYOSIN** interact to generate a muscle contraction

14 - Lifting weights results in hypertrophy of **FAST** twitch muscle fibers

15 - Hereditary disorder of defective osteoclasts leading to bone overgrowth
OSTEOPETROSIS. *Increased bone density so known as "marble bone disease."*

19 - Your patient with sickle cell has osteomyelitis, so be sure to consider this bug (genus)
SALMONELLA

21 - If you have bad proline and lysine hydroxylation, you may be suffering from **SCURVY**

Down:

1 - Slipped **CAPITAL** femoral epiphysis
SCFE typically presents with a painful limp between 7 and 11 years of age; more common in boys.

2 - Gap junctions are present in this type of muscle fibers
SMOOTH

3 - Osgood–Schlatter disease is knee pain in an active teenager resulting from partial avulsion of this tuberosity
TIBIAL

5 - Blue sclerae: Osteogenesis **IMPER-FECTA**

7 - Tick-borne disease that can cause arthritis
LYME

8 - Calcium binds to **CALMODULIN** to activate myosin light-chain kinase
Thankfully, no patient ever comes in saying their calmodulin is acting up.

9 - To start the process of skeletal muscle contraction, action potentials cause **DEPOLARIZATION** of T-tubules

12 - Dry eyes, dry mouth, arthritis just might be this syndrome
SJOGREN'S

16 - Type 1 muscle fibers are **SLOW** twitch

17 - "Onion skin" appearance in bones:
EWING'S sarcoma

18 - Sarcomere separators
Z-LINES

20 - Binds to myosin head and releases actin (acronym)
ATP. *Turns out this stuff is kind of important.*

35 Your Nephrolithiasis Test Came Back...*

Yemeng Lu

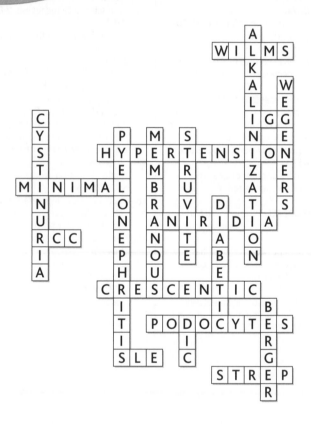

*...unfortunately, you didn't pass.

Across:

2 - Histologic examination of a mass shows embryonic glomerular structures in a spindle-cell stroma in a patient with chromosome 11 mutations; this suggests **WILM'S** tumor

5 - Linear deposits of **IgG** along the basement membrane = Goodpasture syndrome
Circulating IgG antibodies are directed against an antigen intrinsic to the glomerular basement membrane.

9 - Renal biopsy shows reduplication of the elastic lamina and fibrosis of the media of the arcuate arteries; the patient most likely has **HYPERTENSION**
Benign nephrosclerosis can develop in hypertensive patients.

10 - **MINIMAL** change disease on electron microscopy shows podocyte effacement
It is the most frequent cause of nephrotic syndrome in children.

12 - "A" in WAGR complex stands for **ANIRIDIA**
WAGR = Wilm's tumor, Aniridia, Genitourinary anomalies, and mental Retardation.

13 - Overgrowth of renal polygonal clear cells filled with lipids and carbohydrates lead to (acronym)
RCC. Clear cell carcinomas are a type of renal cell carcinoma.

14 - Goodpasture syndrome, Wegener's granulomatosis, and microscopic polyangiitis can all result in **CRESCENTIC** glomerulonephritis

16 - The visceral layer of the Bowman's capsule is consistent of these cells **PODOCYTES**. *They are visceral epithelial cells that wrap around the capillaries of the glomerulus.*

18 - Patient with skin rash and bilateral arthritis of the knee also has RBC casts on urine analysis, most likely has **SLE** (acronym)
Systemic lupus erythematosus.

19 - Acute post-**STREP** (short form) glomerulonephritis has immune complex deposition humps located subepithelially in the glomerulus

Down:

1 - Treatment for cystine kidney stones involves **ALKALINIZATION** of the urine
Cystine solubility increases by up to threefold in an alkaline urine.

3 - Triad of necrotizing granulomas of the upper airways, renal disease, and vasculitis = **WEGENER'S** granulomatosis

4 - An 8-year-old boy with hexagonal crystals in his urine and a positive nitroprusside cyanide test of the urine has **CYSTINURIA**
It is caused by defective renal tubules that cannot resorb amino acid cysteine.

6 - Kidney at autopsy shows purulent inflammation and accumulation of pus in the renal pelvis; the patient most likely died from **PYELONEPHRITIS**

7 - Type of glomerulonephritis with "spike and dome" appearance on electron microscopy showing subepithelial deposits **MEMBRANOUS**

8 - A woman with neurogenic bladder presenting with an indwelling catheter is found to have a 3-cm stone filling the renal pelvis, most likely composed of **STRUVITE**
Staghorn calculi are associated with infection by urea-splitting bacteria and are composed of magnesium ammonium phosphate (struvite).

11 - Kimmelstiel–Wilson lesion = **DIABETIC** nephropathy

15 - A man with a recent upper respiratory tract infection also has microscopic hematuria, most likely has **BERGER** disease
Berger disease (IgA nephropathy) can develop after respiratory infections.

17 - A woman with retained products of conception dies from **DIC** (acronym) and autopsy shows ischemic necrosis of both kidney cortices
Diffuse cortical necrosis is seen in the setting of disseminated intravascular coagulation.

36 Private Parts Path

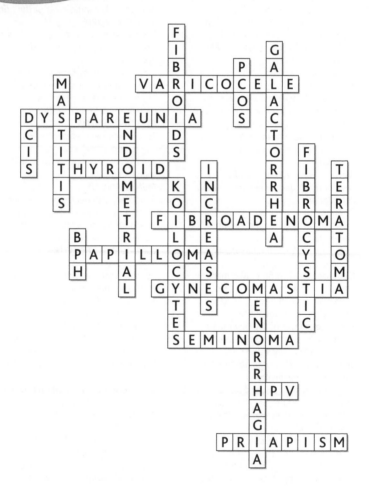

Across:

5 - Dilated veins of the pampiniform plexus, more common on the left **VARICOCELE**. *Varicose veins of the testicles; reason for being more common on the left is because of the drainage at 90-degree angle into the left renal vein.*

6 - Painful intercourse **DYSPAREUNIA**. *Can be a symptom of infection, endometriosis, vaginal atrophy, and so on.*

9 - Struma ovarii contains tissue that can produce this hormone **THYROID**

13 - Small, mobile, firm breast mass in a young woman that increases in tenderness with menstruation is most likely this benign tumor **FIBROADENOMA**

15 - Bloody nipple discharge suggests intraductal **PAPILLOMA** *Always investigate bloody discharge.*

16 - Men on spironolactone might complain of "growing breasts"; the medical term is **GYNECOMASTIA** *Eplerenone is a nonbreast-producing alternative.*

18 - Most common testicular tumor **SEMINOMA**

19 - Virus associated with cervical cancer (acronym) **HPV**. *Human papillomavirus; there is now a vaccine.*

20 - When the Viagra commercial warns of a painful erection lasting more than 4 hours, it is referring to this condition **PRIAPISM**. *(Ouch) More common in sickle cell patients.*

Down:

1 - Common name for leiomyomata of the uterus **FIBROIDS**

2 - Milky nipple discharge **GALACTORRHEA**. *Think prolactinoma.*

3 - Amenorrhea (and infertility), hirsutism, obesity: Clues to this (acronym) **PCOS**. *Polycystic ovarian syndrome.*

4 - Infection of the breast that can lead to abscess **MASTITIS**

6 - Early breast malignancy that has not invaded basement membrane (acronym) **DCIS**. *Ductal carcinoma in situ; found by screening mammogram.*

7 - This cancer is the most common GYN malignancy **ENDOMETRIAL**. *A postmenopausal woman with vaginal bleeding needs an endometrial biopsy.*

8 - This "disease" is a common cause of breast lumps in young women **FIBROCYSTIC**

10 - Prolonged estrogen exposure (increases/decreases) risk of breast cancer **INCREASES**. *(Sorry the puzzle didn't help differentiate the "de-" from the "in-", but we can't make them too easy.)*

11 - Ovarian germ cell tumor; it is pretty freaky because it may contain teeth and hair **TERATOMA**. *Also called dermoid cyst.*

12 - Cells of cervical dysplasia **KOILOCYTES**

14 - Common cause of urinary outflow symptoms in older men (acronym) **BPH**. *Benign prostatic hyperplasia.*

17 - Abnormally heavy menstrual bleeding **MENORRHAGIA**. *Anovulation is a common cause. Metrorrhagia is irregularly timed bleeding (metro = time); there is also menometrorrhagia—you guessed it—frequent and heavy.*

37 This Puzzle May Take You a Lung Time

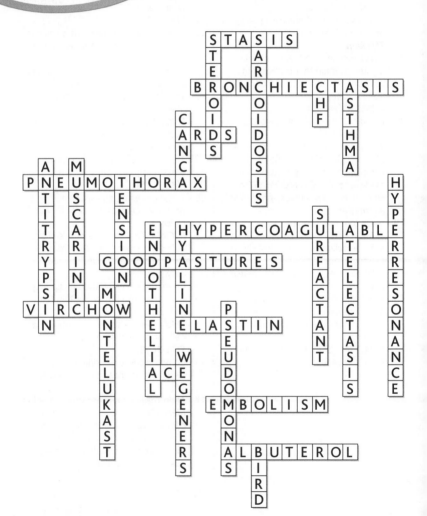

Across:

1 - Clotting triad 1/3: Venous *STASIS*
Often caused by immobility which may occur with illness, injury, hospitalization. May also be a result of mechanical obstruction (indwelling catheter, external vascular compression by an anatomic structure such as a tumor).

3 - Recurrent infections in patients with cystic fibrosis may develop this condition of chronically dilated bronchioles
BRONCHIECTASIS

7 - Severe lung injury resulting from a variety of causes, commonly severe infection and systemic inflammatory disorders (acronym)
ARDS. Adult respiratory distress syndrome.

10 - This may occur spontaneously in tall, thin adolescent and young adult men
PNEUMOTHORAX

15 - Clotting triad 3/3: **HYPERCOAGULABLE** state
Such as pregnancy, cancer, oral contraceptives to name a few.

17 - Another pulmonary–renal syndrome; this disease is caused by antibodies to basement membrane
GOODPASTURE'S. Affects middle aged men usually.

19 - Eponym of clotting triad
VIRCHOW('S)

21 - This protein is degraded in excess in the disease described in #8 down
ELASTIN. Alpha-1-antitrypsin inhibits the enzyme elastase which breaks down elastin. Thus, in the absence of a1-antitrypsin, elastase is uninhibited and destroys elastase, contributing to decreased elasticity of various tissues, including the lungs.

23 - Levels of this enzyme may be increased in #2 down (acronym)
ACE. Angiotensin-converting enzyme.

24 - Pulmonary **EMBOLISM**: Possible cause of sudden death in patients with #19 across
Usually from a deep vein thrombosis in the lower extremity.

25 - Probably the most widely used inhaled, short-acting beta2-agonist
ALBUTEROL

Down:

1 - This drug class exerts its anti-inflammatory effects via inhibition of leukotriene synthesis
STEROIDS. Inhaled steroids are often used as maintenance or controller therapy. Systemic steroids are mostly restricted to use in acute exacerbations.

2 - A systemic disease pathologically characterized by the presence of noncaseating granulomas
SARCOIDOSIS. Typically affects women and African Americans of middle age. Other manifestations include arthritis, erythema nodosum, hypercalcemia, uveitis and, neuropathy.

4 - Fluid-filled alveoli may be the result of this clinical entity (acronym)
CHF. Congestive heart failure. Increased left ventricular pressures transmit back to the pulmonary capillaries and increased hydrostatic pressure causes fluid to leak out.

5 - Many people carry around metered dose inhalers of the drug in #25 across for its rapid effects in treating attacks of this common disease
ASTHMA. Asthma is a disease of hyper-reactivity of the airways. Bronchial smooth muscles constriction eventually leads to muscular hypertrophy and ongoing irritants lead to airway edema and inflammation.

6 - Antibody seen in #22 down (acronym)
CANCA. Cytoplasmic antineutrophil cytoplasmic antibody. Wegener's is one of the "ANCA-associated vasculitides" including microscopic polyangiitis, Churg–Strauss syndrome, and some cases of polyarteritis nodosa.

8 - You might suspect deficiency of the enzyme alpha-1-**ANTITRYPSIN** in a young patient with COPD and liver disease
An autosomal recessive disease.

9 - Ipratropium prevents bronchoconstriction by antagonism of this receptor
MUSCARINIC. An inhaled bronchodilator often used in conjunction with beta2-agonists such as albuterol.

11 - If a one-way valve mechanism is present, you may develop a **TENSION** pneumothorax
Pressure gradually builds in the pleural space, eventually leading to vascular compromise of the great vessels, and death if pressure is unrelieved.

12 - This finding, on physical examination, is characteristic of #10 across
HYPERRESONANCE. Appreciated by percussion of the chest wall.

13 - Deficiency of this molecule leads to the neonatal equivalent of #7 across
SURFACTANT. Seen in prematurity, as lungs do not yet produce surfactant, a molecule which lowers alveolar surface tension and helps alveoli remain open.

14 - Clotting triad 2/3: **ENDOTHELIAL** injury
As occurs postoperatively, or in systemic inflammatory disorders such as infection, rheumatologic disease.

15 - Formation of these pathologic "membranes" is associated with #7 across and #13 down
HYALINE

16 - Collapsed or unexpanded lung tissue
ATELECTASIS

18 - This drug is a leukotriene receptor antagonist
MONTELUKAST. Used in asthma treatment.

20 - This bug often chronically colonizes and recurrently infects patients with cystic fibrosis
PSEUDOMONAS

22 - A rare pulmonary–renal syndrome; the patient may be a young male presenting with bleeding from the upper and lower respiratory tracts and granulomas
WEGENER'S. Wegener's granulomatosis or granulomatosis with polyangiitis is an autoimmune small-medium vessel vasculitis.

26 - Certain types of hypersensitivity pneumonitis may be due to exposure to antigens from this animal
BIRD. Also known as Bird Fancier's Lung or Pigeon-Breeder's Lung. These patients seldom get rid of their birds.

38 Clinical Scramble

ANEWJAY
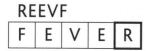
| J | A | N | **E** | W | A | Y |

NOSESIL
| L | E | S | **I** | O | N | S |

REEVF
| F | E | V | E | **R** |

DRACCIA
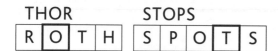
| **C** | A | R | **D** | **I** | **A** | **C** |

RUMMUR
| M | U | R | M | U | R |

THOR
| R | **O** | T | H |

STOPS
| S | P | O | **T** | S |

LORES
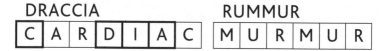
| O | **S** | L | E | R |

SONDE
| **N** | O | **D** | E | S |

ANSWER: **ENDOCARDITIS**

Notes

39 Bug Killers

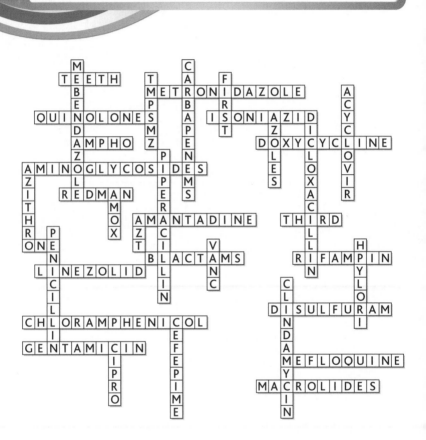

Across:

3 - Use of tetracyclines in childhood may cause discoloration of these
   TEETH. *Hence they are contraindicated in children.*

6 - Used for the treatment of anaerobic infections and protozoa
   METRONIDAZOLE

8 - DNA synthesis inhibitors, used for gram-negative infections
   (FLUORO-)QUINOLONES. *Generally all end in "-floxacin."*

9 - This antibiotic must be given with pyridoxine to prevent neurotoxicity
   ISONIAZID. *Used for the treatment of tuberculosis.*

12 - This "terrible" drug works well for fungal infections (short form)
   AMPHO(TERICIN B). *Forms pores in the fungal (and human) cell membranes.*

13 - Treatment of choice for most tick-borne illness
   DOXYCYCLINE. *Including Lyme, Rocky Mountain Spotted Fever, Ehrlichiosis.*

15 - Irreversibly bind the 30S ribosome
   AMINOGLYCOSIDES. *Includes gentamicin, tobramycin.*

16 - Quick infusion of vancomycin may result in this syndrome (two words)
   RED MAN. *Not a true allergy. Solution is to simply slow the infusion.*

18 - Developed for influenza A, but also useful for Parkinson disease
   AMANTADINE. *Mostly of historical interest, as it is not really used for either indication anymore.*

19 - ***THIRD*** generation cephalosporins: Good gram-negative coverage, weaker gram-positive
   Includes ceftriaxone, cefpodoxime, cefixime, ceftazadime.

21 - Percent of allergic cross-sensitivity between penicillins and cephalosporins
   ONE. *Although you probably were taught that this number is 10%, which is a myth. In fact, the cross-sensitivity between pencillins and 3rd/4th generation cephalosporins approaches 0%.*

24 - Class that inhibits cell wall synthesis (initial the first word)
   B(ETA) LACTAMS. *Include penicillins, cephalosporins, monobactams, and carbapenems.*

25 - Drug used in prophylaxis for contacts of meningococcal cases
   RIFAMPIN. *Also used in the treatment of Mycobacterial infections.*

26 - Only oral agent with no MRSA resistance
   LINEZOLID. *Very expensive, use generally restricted to MRSA infections.*

28 - Metronidazole may cause a ***DISULFURAM***-like reaction when combined with alcohol

29 - Rarely used agent, associated with aplastic anemia and gray baby syndrome
   CHLORAMPHENICOL. *One remaining indication is treatment of tick-borne illness in patients allergic to doxycycline.*

31 - Great gram-negative and Pseudomonas coverage, but nasty effects on hearing and kidneys
   GENTAMICIN

33 - Antimalarial known for CNS side effects
   MEFLOQUINE

34 - Bind the 23S RNA of the 50S ribosome
   MACROLIDES. *Includes erythromycin, azithromycin.*

Down:

1 - Antihelminthic, useful for variety of worm infestations
   MEBENDAZOLE

2 - Class of "biggest guns" cover all bugs except MRSA
   CARBAPENEMS

4 - Antibiotic associated with Stevens–Johnson syndrome (acronym)
   TMP-SMZ. *Trimethoprim-sulfamethoxazole.*

5 - ____ generation cephalosporins: Good gram-positive coverage, weak gram-negative
   FIRST. *Includes cefazolin, cephalexin.*

7 - Guanosine analog, inhibits viral DNA polymerase, useful for herpes viruses
   ACYCLOVIR

10 - Class of antifungals that inhibit ergosterol synthesis
   AZOLES. *Includes fluconazole, clotrimazole.*

11 - Oral B-lactam that covers *S. aureus*, but NOT MRSA
   DICLOXACILLIN. *Unlike other penicillins, it (along with nafcillin and oxacillin) is not inactivated by B-lactamases.*

14 - B-lactam with Pseudomonas coverage
   PIPERACILLIN. *Usually paired with the B-lactamase inhibitor tazobactam.*

15 - Frequently used in concert with ceftriaxone to provide "atypical" coverage in pneumonia (first three syllables)
   AZITHRO(MYCIN). *Atypicals which may include Mycoplasma, Chlamydia, Legionella spp.*

17 - B-lactam with added activity to gram-negative rods:
   AMOX-icillin
   Makes it useful in the treatment of some UTIs.

18 - Antiretroviral drug used to prevent maternal–fetal HIV transmission (acronym)
   AZT. *Azidothymidine.*

20 - Still works great for Group A Streptococcus and syphilis
   PENICILLIN. *Most other bugs have at least moderate rates of resistance.*

22 - Best bet for MRSA treatment: ***VANC***-omycin
   Nearly all other drugs have some variable levels of resistance.

23 - Amoxicillin, clarithromycin, and metronidazole: A triple therapy for this bug
   H(ELICOBACTER) PYLORI. *Now recognized as a leading cause of peptic ulcer disease.*

27 - Covers gram-positive, anaerobes, and some MRSA, but high association with *C. difficile* superinfection
   CLINDAMYCIN. *Belongs to a class nearly all in its own called lincosamides.*

30 - Broadest spectrum cephalosporin, covers Pseudomonas as well
   CEFEPIME. *The only "fourth generation" cephalosporin.*

32 - Young female with spontaneous Achilles tendon rupture may be on this drug for her UTI (short form)
   CIPRO(FLOXACIN)

40 BuzzWards

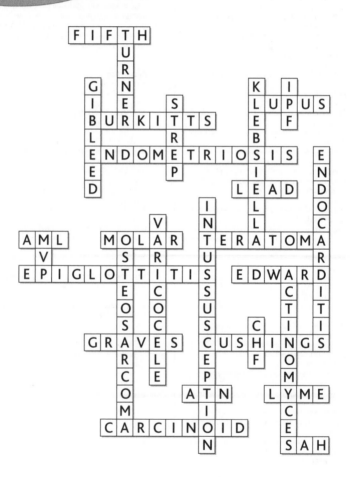

Across:

1 - Slapped cheek (**_FIFTH_** disease)
   Aka Erythema infectiosum, caused by erythrovirus.

7 - Butterfly rash
   LUPUS. *But nearly anything can be a sign of lupus.*

8 - Starry sky B-cells
   BURKITT'S *(lymphoma). Often related to infection with Epstein-Barr virus, and in HIV patients.*

9 - Chocolate cyst
   ENDOMETRIOSIS. *Large cysts containing blood that when coagulated, looks like chocolate.*

11 - Basophilic stippling (toxin)
   LEAD

14 - Auer rods (acronym)
   AML. *Acute myeloid leukemia.*

16 - "Bunch of grapes" or "snowstorm" on ultrasound (**_MOLAR_** pregnancy)
   Hydatidiform mole. May be "complete" (diploid, no embryo) or "partial" (triploid, embryo present).

18 - Neoplasm with teeth
   TERATOMA. *More common in children.*

19 - Thumb sign
   EPIGLOTTITIS. *Seen on lateral x-ray of the neck. The "thumb" is the swollen epiglottis.*

20 - Rocker bottom feet (**_EDWARD_** syndrome)
   Trisomy 18.

23 - Exophthalmos
   GRAVES *(disease)*

24 - Buffalo hump
   CUSHING'S. *Most commonly iatrogenic (i.e., exogenous steroid use).*

25 - Muddy brown casts (acronym)
   ATN. *Acute tubular necrosis; most common cause is ischemia, but may be due to drugs and toxins as well.*

26 - Bull's eye rash
   LYME. *Caused by Borrelia burgdorferi, transmitted by Ixodes tick.*

27 - Flushing and diarrhea
   CARCINOID. *Most common tumor of the appendix; Increased 5-HIAA in urine.*

28 - Worst headache of my life (acronym)
   SAH. *Subarachnoid hemorrhage. Do not miss it!*

Down:

2 - Shield chest (**_TURNER_** syndrome)
   45XO. Other manifestations include short stature, webbed neck, amenorrhea, lack of secondary sex traits, and coarctation.

3 - Coffee ground emesis (acronym)
   GI BLEED, *upper. Coffee grounds suggestive of old blood, not an active bleed.*

4 - Currant jelly sputum (bug)
   KLEBSIELLA. *Often seen in alcoholics who aspirate.*

5 - Honeycomb lung (acronym)
   IPF. *Idiopathic pulmonary fibrosis.*

6 - Strawberry tongue (bug, short form)
   STREP. *Manifestation of scarlet fever due to Group A streptococcus infection.*

10 - Splinter hemorrhages
   ENDOCARDITIS. *An embolic phenomenon.*

12 - Currant jelly stool
   INTUSSUSCEPTION. *May be seen in association with Henoch–Schonlein purpura.*

13 - Bag of worms
   VARICOCELE. *More common in the L scrotum as the L testicular vein drains to the L renal vein at a 90-degree angle, whereas the R testicular vein drains to the IVC.*

15 - Midsystolic click (acronym)
   MVP. *Mitral valve prolapse. Most common valve disorder, seen in young women commonly.*

17 - Sunburst on bone x-ray
   OSTEOSARCOMA. *And development of Codman triangle.*

21 - Sulfur granules (bug)
   ACTINOMYCES. *Most commonly affecting head and neck, often confused with a mass.*

22 - Nutmeg liver (underlying cause, acronym)
   CHF. *Liver injury caused by chronic R-sided congestive heart failure, causing impaired venous return and chronic hepatic congestion.*

41 Out Damned Spot!

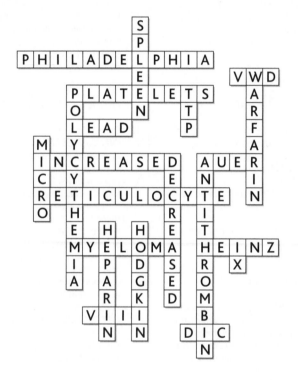

Across:

2 - t(9:22) results in **PHILADELPHIA** chromosome which results in leukemia
Chronic myelogenous (CML).

3 - Most common hereditary bleeding disorder (acronym)
vWD. *Von Willebrand Disease due to decreased vWF, leading to defect in intrinsic pathway.*

5 - ITP is due to antibodies against these **PLATELETS.** *Idiopathic thrombocytopenic purpura.*

7 - Basophilic stippling seen in **LEAD** toxicity

9 - #12 across count is (increased/ decreased) in hemolytic anemia
INCREASED. *Bone marrow is trying to catch up.*

11 - Rods seen in acute myeloblastic leukemia
AUER

12 - Nonnucleated immature RBC formed in bone marrow
RETICULOCYTE

15 - Lytic lesions on plain x-ray, think multiple **MYELOMA**
See the M-spike on serum protein electrophoresis due to too much gamma-globulin.

16 - These bodies are seen in G6PD deficiency (hint: Ketchup and 57)
HEINZ. *Due to oxidation of iron; according to their website, Heinz is the most global of all US-based food companies.*

18 - Hemophilia A is the deficiency of factor **VIII** (Roman numeral)

19 - A severely ill patient with elevated level of fibrin split products, elevated D-dimer, and low level of fibrinogen has this (acronym)
DIC. *Disseminated intravascular coagulation; use up all the clotting factors which leads to bleeding.*

Down:

1 - If you are missing this, you might have Howell–Jolly bodies in your peripheral blood smear
SPLEEN. *Can also be seen if spleen just does not work well.*

4 - Follow the INR (a reflection of PT) to assess effect of this drug
WARFARIN. *Subtherapeutic INR diminishes benefit in preventing thrombosis; supratherapeutic INR increases bleeding risk.*

5 - Increased RBC mass could be **POLYCYTHEMIA** vera

6 - Low platelets, anemia, fever, renal failure, and neurologic changes, think this (acronym)
TTP. *Thrombotic thrombocytopenic purpura. May see schistocytes on smear.*

8 - Iron deficiency anemia is **MICRO**-cytic
Other microcytic anemias include sideroblastosis, anemia of chronic disease, and thalassemia.

10 - Ristocetin aggregation is (increased/ decreased) in vWF deficiency
DECREASED

11 - #13 down binds to **ANTITHROMBIN**-III

13 - Monitor aPTT to assess the effect of this drug
HEPARIN

14 - Reed–Sternberg cells seen in **HODGKIN** disease
Binucleate look like owl eyes.

17 - Hemophilia B is the deficiency of factor **IX** (Roman numeral)

42 Doc, I Think It's My Connective Tissue

Across:

3 - One of the DMARDs
METHOTREXATE

5 - Anti-**SMITH** antibodies are highly specific for lupus
Anti-dsDNA antibodies are also very specific; ANA are sensitive but not very specific.

6 - A child with bowed legs and thin skull bones probably has ____
RICKETS. *Caused by vitamin D deficiency.*

7 - One of the 6Ps of compartment syndrome
PALLOR. *Others are pain, paresthesias, paralysis, pulseless, poikilothermic.*

8 - Boutonniere deformity is usually seen in this type of arthritis
RHEUMATOID

9 - Classic rash of lupus
MALAR

11 - Uric acid crystals in joints
GOUT. *Crystals are needle-shaped and negatively birefringent.*

12 – **HLA**-B27
Stands for human leukocyte antigen.

15 - TB of the spine: **POTT** disease
Some say Pott's disease.

17 - It is the R in CREST syndrome
RAYNAUD'S. *Calcinosis, Raynaud disease, esophageal dysmotility, sclerodactyly, Telangiectasia.*

19 - A primary bone malignancy
OSTEOSARCOMA

20 - Calcium pyrophosphate crystal deposition in joints
PSEUDOGOUT. *Crystals are positively birefringent.*

22 - A patient with dry eyes, dry mouth, and arthritis may have **SJOGREN'S** syndrome

23 - Beethoven, who had a prominent forehead and hearing loss, might have had this disease of abnormal bone activity.
PAGET'S. *The hearing loss results from narrowing of the auditory foramen.*

24 - Noncaseating granulomatous disease
SARCOIDOSIS. *Most common in African-American women.*

Down:

1 - Heliotrope rash is classic for
DERMATOmyositis

2 - Conjunctivitis, urethritis, and arthritis:
REITER'S syndrome
Mnemonic is "can't see, can't pee, can't climb a tree."

4 - #12 across is associated with **ANKYLOSING** spondylitis
AS is one of the spondyloarthropathies.

7 - Gout of the big toe
PODAGRA

10 - Most common cause of dwarfism
ACHONDROPLASIA

13 - Allopurinol, a treatment for gout, inhibits **XANTHINE** oxidase

14 - "Marble bones"
OSTEOPETROSIS

16 - Condition of decreased bone density
OSTEOPOROSIS. *Osteopenia is also decreased bone density but that has not reached the level to be called osteoporosis.*

18 - "Sausage fingers"
DACTYLITIS. *Can be seen in psoriatic arthritis.*

21 - A type of aggressive sarcoma, mostly affecting young boys
EWING'S. *Associated with 11;22 translocation.*

43 Clues in a Drug's Name

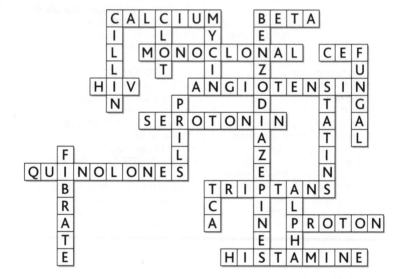

Across:

1 - The "-dipines" are the dihydropyridine form of these channel blockers
CALCIUM. *For example, amlodipine. Nondihydropyridines are verapamil and diltiazem.*

4 - If a drug ends in -olol, there is a good chance it blocks these receptors
BETA. *For example, propranolol, metoprolol, atenolol; can be cardioselective.*

5 - "-mabs" are **MONOCLONAL** antibodies

6 - You will find these three letters in the names of many cephalosporins
CEF

8 - If your patient is on a drug ending in -avir, -udine, or both, he probably has this infection (acronym)
HIV

9 - Drugs that block this receptor (the type II AT1) end in –sartan
ANGIOTENSIN. *For example, candesartan, losartan.*

12 - Drugs ending in -etine or -opram block reuptake of this
SEROTONIN. *For example, fluoxetine, citalopram.*

14 - "-floxacins" are this class of antibiotics
QUINOLONES. *For example, levofloxacin, ciprofloxacin.*

15 - Medications for acute migraine
TRIPTANS. *For example, sumatriptan.*

17 - Drugs that block this pump often end in -prazole
PROTON. *For example, omeprazole, rabeprazole.*

18 - Drugs ending in -tidine, like ranitidine, block these receptors
HISTAMINE

Down:

1 - Drugs ending in this inhibit mucopeptide synthesis in the bacterial cell wall
CILLIN. *Classic is penicillin.*

2 - If you are calling stat for a drug ending in -plase, you are probably trying to break up one of these somewhere (Useless hint: Not a fight)
CLOT. *Can be for myocardial infarction or stroke.*

3 - Macrolides often end in these five letters
MYCIN. *For example, azithromycin or clarithromycin.*

4 - These typically end in -lam or –pam
BENZODIAZEPINES. *For example, diazepam or alprazolam.*

7 - "-azoles" are anti-**FUNGAL**
Not to be confused with the -prazoles, as in #17 across.

10 - HMG-CoA reductase inhibitors
STATINS

11 - ACE inhibitors
PRILS

13 - Drugs with this ending help lower triglycerides
FIBRATE

15 - A "-triptyline" is one of this class of drugs (acronym)
TCA. *Tricyclic antidepressant, sometimes used for other indications capitalizing on their anticholinergic effects.*

16 - Drugs ending in -azosin block peripheral **ALPHA** receptors
Doxazosin, for example, which is useful in BPH.

44 What is the Most Common...?

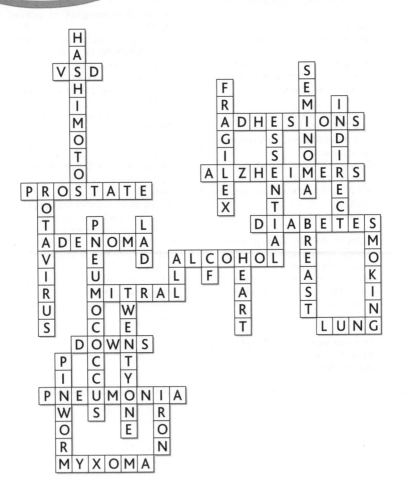

Across:

2 - Congenital heart defect (acronym)
   VSD. *Ventricular septal defect. May be membranous or muscular. The former is the more common. A noncyanotic lesion.*

6 - Cause of intestinal obstruction
   ADHESIONS. *Usually due to scarring from prior surgeries.*

8 - Cause of dementia
   ALZHEIMER'S

9 - Cancer in men
   PROSTATE

13 - Cause of chronic kidney disease
   DIABETES

16 - Cause of primary hyperparathyroidism
   ADENOMA. *Usually benign.*

17 - Cause of cirrhosis
   ALCOHOL

20 - Valve affected by rheumatic fever
   MITRAL. *Causes mitral valve stenosis, and a fish-mouth appearance.*

22 - Cause of cancer death
   LUNG. *And the second most common overall cancer in men and women.*

23 - Chromosomal disorder (**DOWN'S** syndrome)
   TRISOMY 21.

25 - Cause of death in Alzheimer patients
   PNEUMONIA

27 - Cancer of the heart
   MYXOMA. *A benign tumor, with characteristic "ball valve" mechanism.*

Down:

1 - Cause of hypothyroidism
   HASHIMOTO'S. *Most common autoimmune disease overall as well.*

3 - Cancer of the testes
   SEMINOMA

4 - Heritable cause of mental retardation
   FRAGILE X

5 - Type of hernia
   INDIRECT. *Lateral to the inferior epigastric artery. Direct hernias are medial.*

7 - Form of hypertension
   ESSENTIAL. *Meaning without an identifiable secondary cause.*

10 - Bug causing diarrhea in children
   ROTAVIRUS

11 - Bug in community-acquired pneumonia
   PNEUMOCOCCUS. *Aka S. pneumoniae.*

12 - Artery for MI (acronym)
   LAD. *Left anterior descending, aka "the widow maker."*

14 - Cancer in women
   BREAST

15 - Preventable cause of death
   SMOKING. *Accounts for nearly half a million preventable deaths each year.*

17 - Cause of leukemia in young children (acronym)
   ALL. *Acute lymphoblastic leukemia. Usually responsive to therapy with good prognosis.*

18 - Fatal genetic disease in Caucasians (acronym)
   CF. *Cystic fibrosis, although many patients now live well into adulthood.*

19 - Cause of death in US (organ)
   HEART. *Specifically, ischemic heart disease.*

21 - Cause of congenital adrenal hyperplasia (**TWENTY-ONE**-hydroxylase deficiency)
   Think of this in a newborn with ambiguous genitalia.

24 - Worm infection in US
   PINWORM. *Enterobius vermicularis. Anal pruritis. May be detected by scotch tape test.*

26 - Dietary deficiency
   IRON. *Causes microcytic, hypochromic anemia.*

45 This Puzzle Takes Guts

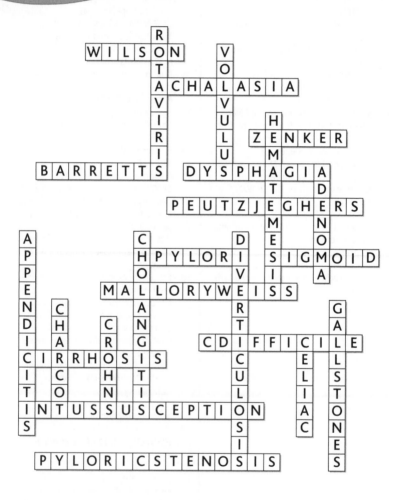

Across:

2 - Kayser–Fleischer rings: **_WILSON_** disease
Due to the deficiency of ceruloplasmin, leading to copper depositions; in this case, in the cornea.

4 - "Bird beak" esophagus (on barium swallow)
ACHALASIA. *LES doesn't relax.*

6 - Pharyngeal pouch in which food can get stuck: **_ZENKER_** diverticulum

7 - Metaplasia in distal esophagus
BARRETTS. *Increased risk for carcinoma.*

8 - Trouble swallowing
DYSPHAGIA. *Causes include scleroderma, achalasia, diffuse esophageal spasm, and obstructing lesion.*

10 - Hamartomas of GI tract and hyperpigmentation: **_PEUTZ–JEGHERS_** syndrome

14 - Duodenal ulcers are associated with this germ (only use first initial of genus)
HPYLORI. *Treatment is a combination of antibiotics and proton-pump inhibition.*

15 - Most common site of colon cancer
SIGMOID

16 - If you drink too much after your Step 1 exam, leading to vomiting that tears your esophagus, it is called a **_MALLORY–WEISS_** tear

20 - Organism responsible for pseudomembranous colitis (only use first initial of genus)
C. DIFFICILE

22 - Antimitochondrial antibodies are seen in primary biliary **_CIRRHOSIS_**

23 - Telescoping intestines
INTUSSUSCEPTION. *Not to be confused with a Leonard DiCaprio movie.*

24 - Two-word diagnosis if you feel an "olive" in the epigastrium of a 2-week-old boy who has been having projectile vomiting
PYLORIC STENOSIS

Down:

1 - Most common cause of diarrhea in infants
ROTAVIRUS

3 - Twisting intestines
VOLVULUS. *(Twisting Intestines would be a cool rock band name).*

5 - Blood in the vomit
HEMATEMESIS. *Usually an upper GI bleed.*

9 - Precancerous colon polyp
ADENOMA. *Hyperplastic polyps are not precancerous.*

11 - Pain at McBurney's point associated with anorexia suggests this diagnosis
APPENDICITIS

12 - #17 down suggests this diagnosis
CHOLANGITIS

13 - Common cause of lower GI bleeding
DIVERTICULOSIS

17 - Fever, jaundice, RUQ pain: **_CHARCOT_** triad

18 - Major cause of acute pancreatitis
GALLSTONES. *Other major causes are alcohol and hypertriglyceridemia.*

19 - Skip lesions in the colon
CROHN'S

21 - Gluten sensitivity: **_CELIAC_** disease

46 A Biased Puzzle?

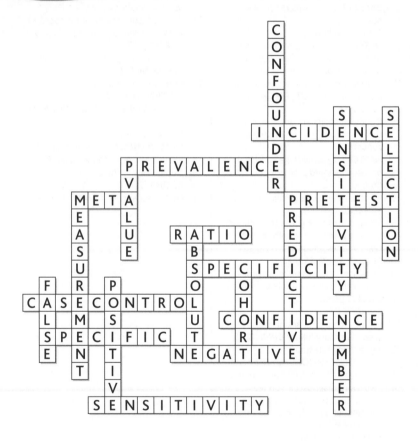

Across:

4 - The proportion of people who develop an outcome over a given time period
INCIDENCE. *And prevalence is the proportion of people who "have" the outcome at a specific time.*

5 - A cross-sectional study is sometimes called a **PREVALENCE** study because it can be used to estimate this

6 - A **META** -analysis is a kind of study that mathematically pools the data from multiple studies to generate a "best" estimate
These may be part of a systematic review, but not all systematic reviews include meta-analysis.

7 - Prevalence of a disease in a population of patients can be used as an estimate of the **PRETEST** probability

8 - The odds of the outcome among the exposed group divided by the odds of the outcome among the nonexposed group is the odds **RATIO**

10 - For a diagnostic test, true negatives divided by true negatives plus false positives
SPECIFICITY

14 - An investigator selects 20 medical students who have step one phobia and 20 students who do not; she then calls them and asks whether they ever did CrossWard puzzles to see if there is an association; this is a **CASE CONTROL** study (two words)
This design is especially susceptible to a form of measurement bias called recall bias.

15 - The interval that represents the range of values expected 95 out of 100 times (if a study is repeated 100 times) is the 95% **CONFIDENCE** interval

17 - A highly **SPECIFIC** test when positive is helpful at ruling in disease
Remember SpPin and SnNout.

18 - The posttest probability of a disease given a negative test is equal to 1 minus the **NEGATIVE** predictive value

19 - Test X detects 97% of disease among people who have the disease; 97% is the **SENSITIVITY**

Down:

1 - In a study that shows gray hair is associated with coronary artery disease, age is a **CONFOUNDER**

2 - For a diagnostic test, true positives divided by true positives plus false negatives
SENSITIVITY

3 - When a lot of people in one group of a study drop out and few in the other group drop out, this is a potential **SELECTION** bias

5 - By convention (and quite arbitrarily), a study's finding is considered statistically significant if this is <0.05
P-VALUE

6 - A study bias in which it is easier to tell if people in one group had the outcome is a differential **MEASUREMENT** bias

7 - For a diagnostic test, true positives divided by all positives: Positive **PREDICTIVE** value

9 - Drug A reduces blood clots by 5% while Drug B reduces blood clots by 2.5%; the **ABSOLUTE** risk reduction is 2.5%

11 - An investigator identifies 800 people free of syndrome Z and follows them over time to see if exposure to energy drinks is associated with development of syndrome Z; this is a **COHORT** study design

12 - The positive test in a patient with a very low pretest probability is likely to be a **FALSE** positive test

13 - The posttest probability of a disease given a positive test is the **POSITIVE** predictive value

16 - The inverse of the absolute risk reduction is the **NUMBER** needed to treat

47 Can You "Crack" this Puzzle?

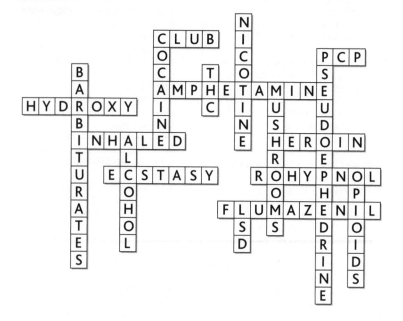

Across:

2 - GHB, ketamine, and roofies are known as "**CLUB** drugs" because of where teenagers use them
3 - Hallucinogen that is NMDA receptor agonist (acronym)
PCP. *Phencyclidine, street name Angel dust.*
6 - Causes increased catecholamine release
AMPHETAMINE. *This is speed.*
8 - Gamma- **HYDROXY** -butyric acid
This is GHB.
9 - Whippets, poppers, and snappers are all taken by this method
INHALED
11 - Street name "smack"
HEROIN
12 - MDMA common name
ECSTASY
13 – "Roofies"
ROHYPNOL. *(Made more famous in The Hangover movie.)*
15 - Used to treat benzodiazepine overdose
FLUMAZENIL

Down:

1 - This can stimulate and relax
NICOTINE. *This is why people who smoke cigarettes do so for all occasions.*
2 - Blocks norepinephrine, dopamine, and serotonin reuptake
COCAINE
3 - This decongestant is no longer available directly on store shelves because it is an ingredient in meth labs
PSEUDOEPHEDRINE
4 - Potentiate GABA's action by keeping chloride channels open
BARBITURATES
5 - Active compound in marijuana (acronym)
THC. *Tetrahydrocannabinol.*
7 - Psilocybin: Street name "magic **MUSHROOMS**" (Hint: Not "Mike")
10 - Withdrawal can lead to delirium tremens
ALCOHOL
14 - Overdose of this class of drugs can cause pinpoint pupils and respiratory depression
OPIOIDS
16 - Withdrawal leads to flashbacks (acronym)
LSD. *Lysergic acid diethylamide.*

48 Clinical Scramble

VEERF

F	E	V	E	R

LOSTKEYOUSIC

L	E	U	K	O	C	Y	T	O	S	I	S

CAPETHANY

T	A	C	H	Y	P	N	E	A

CINTIFONE

I	N	F	E	C	T	I	O	N

IPENNYSHOOT

H	Y	P	O	T	E	N	S	I	O	N

ANSWER: **SEPTIC SHOCK**

Notes

49 This Puzzle is More Fun than a Fungus Ball

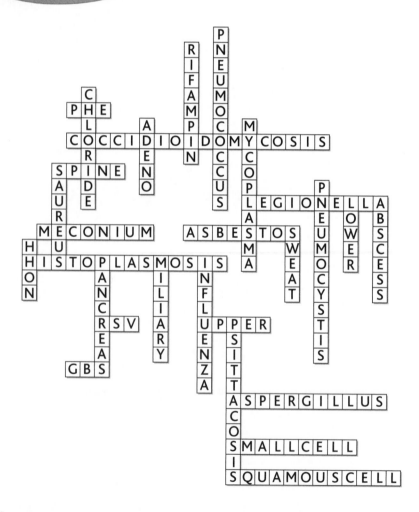

Across:

4 - Deletion of this amino acid, responsible for the most common fatal genetic disease in caucasians (acronym)
PHE. PHENYLALANINE. *Deleted from the CFTR gene at position 508, on chromosome 7.*

7 - Fungal pneumonia seen in the American Southwest
COCCIDIOIDOMYCOSIS. *Caused by Coccidioides immitis, aka Valley Fever.*

8 - Pott disease: Extrapulmonary form of TB that affects the **SPINE**

10 - This atypical pneumonia bug (genus) lives in the water supply and may be associated with outbreaks
LEGIONELLA. *Legionella pneumophila, a gram negative that mostly affects the elderly. Named for an outbreak that occurred at a convention of the American Legion.*

13 - **MECONIUM** ileus: Form of small-bowel obstruction seen in infants, may be a presentation of CF

14 - Exposure to this mineral increases the risk of bronchogenic carcinoma and mesothelioma
ASBESTOS. *Seen in those who have worked in shipbuilding, plumbing, roofing. Histologically identified as a "ferruginous body."*

17 - Fungal infection common in Ohio and Mississippi River Valleys
HISTOPLASMOSIS. *Caused by Histoplasma capsulatum. Usually a subclinical infection, evidenced on x-ray as calcified granuloma.*

21 - This virus causes endless cases of viral pneumonias and bronchiolitis in children during winter months (acronym)
RSV. RESPIRATORY SYNCYTIAL VIRUS.

22 - **UPPER** lobe: Usual site of secondary tuberculosis

24 - Most common cause of pneumonia in a newborn (acronym)
GBS. GROUP B STREPTOCOCCUS. *aka S. agalactiae.*

25 - Fungal infection which may form a fungus ball
ASPERGILLUS

26 - Lung cancer associated with poor prognosis and paraneoplastic syndromes (two words)
SMALL CELL. *aka oat cell, small basophilic cells have neuroendocrine origin. Most common paraneoplastic syndromes results from ACTH and ADH secretion.*

27 - Cancer strongly associated with smoking and in central location (also two words)
SQUAMOUS CELL. *May create paraneoplastic syndrome via secretion of PTH-related peptide.*

Down:

1 - The most common bug causing typical pneumonia (species form)
PNEUMOCOCCUS. *Streptococcus pneumoniae, a gram-positive coccus in pairs.*

2 - Treatment of active TB with this drug may turn your urine orange
RIFAMPIN. *Blocks RNA synthesis via inhibition of RNA polymerase.*

3 - Electrolyte transport affected by #4 across
CHLORIDE. *Decreased ability to secrete chloride into the lumen causes drying and thickening of secretions.*

5 - **ADENO** carcinoma: Most common type of lung cancer
Often associated with smoking, located peripheral.

6 - **MYCOPLASMA** pneumoniae: One of the "atypicals" and the cause of "walking pneumonia"

8 - Secondary infection with this bug may occur in primary infection due to #20 down (initial the genus)
S. AUREUS. *Staphylococcal pneumonia, especially if due to MRSA, may be deadly.*

9 - Life-threatening pneumonia in immuno-compromised patients, especially HIV
PNEUMOCYSTIS. *Caused by the fungus Pneumocystis jiroveci, previously thought to be a protozoan.*

11 - **LOWER** lobe: Usual location of #16 down

12 - Staphylococcal pneumonia may lead to the formation of this cavitary lesion
ABSCESS. *S. aureus in particular is often associated with abscess formation. S. pneumonia may follow a viral infection, particularly influenza.*

15 - **SWEAT** test: Diagnostic test for CF
High levels of sweat chloride are diagnostic.

16 - **GHON** complex: Caseating granuloma seen in primary tuberculosis

18 - Other nonlung organ primarily affected in patients with cystic fibrosis
PANCREAS. *Thus CF may present as nutritional failure to thrive with malabsorptive stools.*

19 - **MILIARY** TB: Tuberculosis outside of the lung

20 - Frequent seasonal mutations require yearly immunizations against this respiratory virus
INFLUENZA

23 - If you get chlamydia from your bird, you might have this
PSITTACOSIS. *Caused by Chlamydia psittaci, not trachomatis.*

50 Step 1 Potpourri

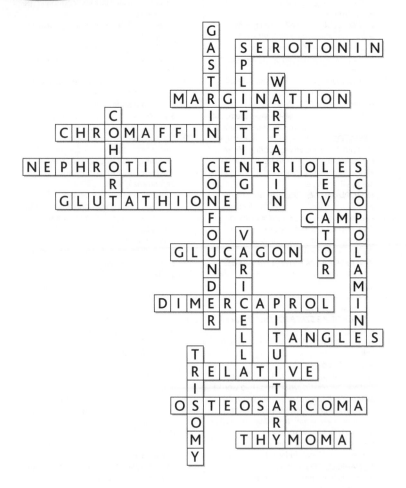

Across:

2 - Mediator released during mast cell activation that directly increases vascular permeability
SEROTONIN

4 - Term for movement of white blood cells to the periphery of the microcirculation
MARGINATION

6 - If you ever see a pheochromocytoma, recall that it is a tumor of these cells in the adrenal medulla
CHROMAFFIN. *(Most likely you will never actually see a patient with a pheo.)*

7 - Proteinuria, edema, hypoalbuminemia, hyperlipidemia: **NEPHROTIC** syndrome
The protein is lost through the kidneys, resulting in proteinuria; the low protein state is reflected in the blood as hypoalbuminemia, and due to loss of osmotic pressure, the patient gets edematous.

8 - Made up of nine tubular triplets, these help with spindle formation
CENTRIOLES. *Kind of sounds like a baseball team – the Los Angeles Centrioles.*

11 - Enzyme that protects red blood cells from in vivo generated hydrogen peroxide: **GLUTATHIONE** peroxidase
We admit this is a tough one.

12 - Cholera infection causes massive diarrhea via a mechanism increasing levels of this in the intestines (acronym)
CAMP

14 - Increases plasma glucose by stimulating glycogenolysis and gluconeogenesis
GLUCAGON

15 - Treatment for lead poisoning
DIMERCAPROL. *(And stop eating lead.)*

17 - Pathologic finding in the hippocampus of patients with Alzheimer disease: neurofibrillary **TANGLES**

19 - Patients taking drug X have a risk of death of 10% while patients taking drug Y have a risk of death of 5%; 50% is the **RELATIVE** risk reduction
And 5% is the absolute risk reduction.

20 - Patients with retinoblastoma are at increased risk of developing this cancer
OSTEOSARCOMA

21 - Tumor associated with myasthenia gravis
THYMOMA

Down:

1 - Zollinger-Ellison syndrome is characterized by overproduction of this
GASTRIN

2 - Defense mechanism in which people or events are seen as entirely good or entirely bad
SPLITTING. *Borderline patients do this classically.*

3 - Anticoagulant reversed by vitamin K
WARFARIN. *It is also rat poison.*

5 - Study design in which subjects are initially free of disease and followed over time to assess whether an exposure is associated with development of disease
COHORT

8 - In a research study, a third factor that is associated with both the exposure and the outcome is called a **CONFOUNDER**

9 - Muscle that raises the soft palate during swallowing: **LEVATOR** veli palatine

10 - Antimuscarinic used to prevent motion sickness
SCOPOLAMINE

13 - Virus that causes shingles when reactivated (genus)
VARICELLA. *VZV – varicella zoster virus.*

16 - Bitemporal hemianopia may signify a tumor in this gland
PITUITARY

18 - Down syndrome: **TRISOMY** 21